The Limits of Principle

The Limits of Principle

Deciding Who Lives and What Dies

Tom Koch

PRAEGER

Westport, Connecticut
London

Library of Congress Cataloging-in-Publication Data

Koch, Tom, 1949–
    The limits of principle : deciding who lives and what dies / Tom
Koch.
      p. cm.
    Includes bibliographical references and index.
    ISBN 0–275–96407–8 (alk. paper)
    1. Medical ethics—Methodology.   2. Allocation of organs, tissues,
etc.—Moral and ethical aspects.   3. Anencephaly—Moral and ethical
aspects. I. Title.
R724.K6   1998
174'.24—dc21   98–23553

British Library Cataloguing in Publication Data is available.

Library of Congress Catalog Card Number: 98–23553
ISBN: 0–275–96407–8

First published in 1998

Praeger Publishers, 88 Post Road West, Westport, CT 06881
An imprint of Greenwood Publishing Group, Inc.

Printed in the United States of America

The paper used in this book complies with the
Permanent Paper Standard issued by the National
Information Standards Organization (Z39.48–1984).

10 9 8 7 6 5 4 3 2 1

Copyright Acknowledgments

The author and publisher are grateful to the following sources for granting permission to reprint
from their materials:

Permission to use materials originally appearing in *Cambridge Quarterly of Healthcare Ethics*, a Cambridge University publication, is gratefully acknowledged by the author.

Permission to use materials originally appearing in *Theoretical Medicine and Bioethics*, a Kluwer Academic publishers journal, is gratefully acknowledged by the author.

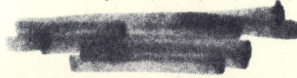

The primary good that we distribute is membership in some human community.

—Michael Walzer, *Spheres of Justice*

Contents

Acknowledgments

This book was born at the 1995 International Conference on Bioethics, Berkeley, California. Invited by Prof. Tommi Kushner, an editor of the *Cambridge Quarterly of Healthcare Ethics*, I left with the conviction that a new and different approach to problems like anencephaly and organ transplant eligibility was required. In my attempts to come to grips with these problems, I was encouraged by Tommi, her fellow CQ editor Dave Thomasma of Loyola University, and their colleague at *Theoretical Medicine and Bioethics*, Dr. Gerrit Kimsma. All provided me with the enviable opportunity to work on parts of these problems through the writing of journal articles, which they and peer reviewers ably critiqued. My understanding was enriched by their suggestions and the opportunity to write in this fashion.

Testing the small focus group approach would have been impossible without the support of persons at The Hospital for Sick Children, Toronto. My appointment as research associate was approved and the work facilitated through the support of Christine Harrison, Ph.D., director of the hospital's Department of Bioethics. Micheline Cox, the department's able administrative assistant, gave the type of logistic support without which no program can survive in a busy urban hospital. My friend and colleague, bioethicist Mary Rowell, championed this work from the start, generously sharing her vast, practical experience as well as her extensive knowledge of medical and bioethical literatures. Finally, hospital psychiatrist Dr. Arlette Lefebvre provided both superb insights and excellent critiques of this work in progress. I am indebted to them all.

I am especially grateful, however, to those persons who took part in the focus groups described in later chapters of this book. Busy staff persons at the hospital took hours out of their hectic schedules to participate in this program. Members of the Niagara Falls Chapter of the Down Syndrome Family Association welcomed me into their homes to discuss these personal, difficult, and sometimes painful issues. My neighbors in Toronto's Beaches community gave up evenings to assure that I would have the community input this work required. It is my hope that, in seeing this book, none will believe their generosity of spirit and time was ill used or abused.

It is also a pleasure to acknowledge the staff at Greenwood Press, my primary publisher for eight years. Dr. James T. Sabin has served as both editor of and advisor to my book writing career. Catherine Lyons, this book's production editor, has supervised the transition of my various manuscripts into finished volumes. Ellen Louer and her predecessor, Denise Van Acker, have ably handled the complex task of book promotion. My thanks to them all.

Finally, I owe a very personal acknowledgment to my friends, Prof. Mark Ridgley, Department of Geography, University of Hawaii, and Prof. Walter Wright the chairperson of Clark University's Department of Philosophy. It was Mark Ridgley who first suggested I consider the Analytic Hierarchy Process (AHP) and then worked with me as I struggled to understand the results it returned in this project. Time and again, Walter Wright answered my questions about ethics and philosophy, suggesting new readings after reviewing early drafts of this work. They helped because we are friends and because both are by nature consummate teachers, people whose delight it is to help others to learn. This book is affectionately dedicated to them both.

1

Deciding Who Lives and Who Dies: Modernity's Context

In November 1962, *Life Magazine* published a ground-breaking article, "They Decide Who Lives, Who Dies,"[1] describing the deliberations of the Seattle, Washington, committee whose members were charged with selecting which patients would gain entry in the city's then new, hemodialysis program. The year before, Dr. Belding Scribner had invented the arteriovenous shunt and cannula that made dialysis possible and with it the potential of continued life for patients with progressive, irreversible kidney disease. By providing an artificial means of cleaning the blood in persons whose own organs could not do the job, Scribner's technology offered hope to thousands of patients with failing kidneys who would die without this treatment.

It quickly became apparent, however, that across the nation many more patients needed dialysis than could be accommodated at the new, expensive, and still rare dialysis centers. Most hospitals created internal committees of physicians to screen applicants for their programs. Seattle, however, took the unusual step of constituting a citizens' committee to define who would receive dialysis and live, and conversely, who would be denied the new treatment and die. Composed of a lawyer, a minister, a banker, a housewife, a state government official, a labor leader, and a surgeon, this group later was called disparagingly the "God Committee."[2]

In its deliberations, the committee reportedly considered criteria ranging from candidate occupation and educational background to community service and family circumstances. While sharply criticized for the use of such social (some would say class-based) data, what distinguished Seattle from other centers was the use of a nonmedical decision-making group, not the criteria committee members used in making their decisions. In rationing hemodyalisis, most centers based their allocative judgments on social criteria such as financial status and employment history. Counterindications leading to candidate rejection at various U.S. hemodialysis centers included, according to one survey in the 1960s, "mental deficiency," a criminal record, an inferior employment history, and indigence.[3]

At one level, the dilemma of hemodialysis was a problem of resource allocation: A congress of potential users required a service unavailable in sufficient quantity to accommodate all potential claimants. The problem, then, was to define a method for choosing between equally needy candidates in a way that was consistent and responsible. Should it be a decision made by medical professionals, by social leaders, by lottery, or by some other procedure? It was also, however, a question of what criteria should be used to distinguish between patients who were socially diverse but all clinically fragile.

Finally, after lengthy debate, the U.S. Congress decided in the early 1970s to fund sufficient dialysis centers to assure treatment of all potential claimants. Indiana Senator Vance Hartke told his colleagues in Congress that a nation able to afford billions of dollars annually on cosmetics and other nonessential items should, "Set our national priorities through a national effort to bring kidney disease treatment within reach of all those in need."[4] When the national program was approved, federal funding removed the limits of scarcity from the arena of dialysis treatment and with it the problem of allocating a scarce but crucial resource. In recent years Congress' largess has resulted in the annual treatment of 150,000 U.S. patients in a program costing approximately $3 billion a year.

Debate over the allocation of scarce health resources did not begin or end with the battle over dialysis. Nor is it necessarily defined by modernity's advancing medical technology. Earlier in this century, for example, the eugenics movement in the United States sought to prevent the birth and limit the medical treatment of "defectives" on the grounds that their continuance (and future maintenance) was economically unsustainable. This was the justification both for forced sterilization,[5] and in some cases, the nontreatment of children born with serious defects.[6] More recently, it was common practice in the 1960s to limit aggressive treatment for the poor at many U.S. hospitals. In 1965, for example, less aggressive treatment was given at a "charity" hospital to, "The dope addict, the known prostitute, the assailant in a crime of violence, the vagrant, the known wife beater and other persons whose moral characters are considered reproachable."[7]

In recent years, Oregon used a series of broadly constituted committees to decide which medical procedures would receive state reimbursement and which would not. Defining finite health dollars as a scarce resource, the Oregon program set up a health services commission to define, with public input, criteria by which medical procedures—and thus claimants—would be excluded from public funding.[8] That this rationing largely affected those who could not afford comprehensive private health insurance was an unsettling fact disturbing to many. Lauded for its populist approach, but criticized for its limits, the Oregon approach has been debated by bioethicists, health economists, and, of course, the people whose lives are affected by the program's conclusions.

If the dilemma of hemodialysis was not the first time medicine and economics clashed on the field of philosophy, it was the first time postmodern technology placed medical decision making upon the national agenda. More recently, organ transplantation has offered the focus for a similar debate: Who among the equally needy will receive the scarce liver, the fragile lung, the necessary heart? In an expanding field of scarcity, the more general problem is health care itself. It, too, is increasingly described as a limited resource that must be rationed among the population and weighted to the most worthy claimants rather than simply the most needy among us. The question is constant and stark: If there is not enough for everyone, who will be left out?

BIOETHICS

The general problem of hemodialysis—who decides who will receive scarce but crucial health resources?—is seen by many as the beginning of modern medical bioethics, the first in what has become a series of debates on the justice and ethics of current methods of medical decision making. A "minor form of moral philosophy practiced within medicine,"[9] bioethics' basic approach from the start has been philosophical, the application of midlevel principles (autonomy, beneficence, nonmalfeasance, justice) to the arena of medical allocation and decision making.[10] While often useful and sometimes enlightening, its principlism has proven generally inadequate in the face of the complex problems presented by advancing medical technologies. As Howard Brody put it, "We have usually tried to resolve these questions through appeals to ethical rights, duties, and consequences. This search for a resolution has proved unsatisfactory."[11] The reason for this is clear. "Empirical studies have suggested that the dominant modes of bioethics analysis may bear little relationship to the ethical reasoning actually used in clinical situations," Susan M. Wolf observes. "These sorts of studies suggest that the analytic method bioethics has embraced, most importantly principlism, is at best a means of *post hoc* rationalization."[12] Simply, there is no generally accepted bioethical methodology except *post hoc* rationalization that will define an acceptable answer to the question who lives and who dies.

In recent years the problem has become ever more urgent as the pace of medical advances has increased. "Legal and moral paradigms are coming under unbearable tension" as technology's potential increases while our ability to define the efficacy of its techniques remains stalled.[13] Modern technology has given us the power to save the most fragile newborn but not the knowledge to decide if every infant's life is worth saving. While we have the ability to maintain for years an adult in a "permanent vegetative state," nobody can say with certainty if this is a boon or merely an expensive gesture to the body of a man or a woman whose essential self has expired. The miraculous capability to transplant organs between persons has created the dilemma of how to choose between respective and equally needy recipients when the demand for those organs far exceeds available supply. It has also given us the conundrum of "beating heart donors," persons who while physically alive at one level may be considered dead for the purposes of organ "harvesting."

In the same vein, recent advances in genetic testing allow us to predict the onset of a host of diseases. These advances do not, however, tell us whether the potential of a future illness is sufficient reason to abort a pregnancy or to let a young person die. Knowing an infant will be born with Down syndrome, spina bifida, or a cleft palate does not necessarily mean they should be terminated before birth. Put another way, the knowledge that a fetus will, if it survives, someday develop Huntington's chorea, familial Alzheimer's disease, or breast cancer is one type of fact. Deciding whether that means those potential lives should be eliminated from the human tree demands another type of thinking.

These are what Harvard biologist R. C. Lewontin calls the hard questions of modern medical science, ones simultaneously defining and changing the social context in which medical science itself is utilized.[14] Most questions can be seen, at least in part, as problems of resource allocation: Who will receive the scarce but valuable benefits of medical technology, how will they be distributed, and who will fund them? Certainly, the age-old "sanctity of human life" doctrine's argument for the positive value of even restricted life is no longer strong enough to allow a reflexively inclusive answer to these issues. "Like cosmology before Copernicus," exalts bioethicist Peter Singer, "the traditional doctrine of the sanctity of human life is today in deep trouble."[15] As a result, we are inconsistent and unsure in the realm of medical ethics and its midlevel principles. We praise the vision of Nobel Prize–winning author, Kenzaburo Oe, whose inspiration has been the life of his composer son, Hikari—born with cognitive deficits—while arguing for genetic screening and the subsequent elimination of "defective" persons.[16] At one level we embrace the insight of neurologist Oliver Sacks,[17] a principle investigator into atypical humanity, while simultaneously advancing a modern vision of eugenics,[18] one that says a restricted life is no life at all.

CURRENT CONTEXTS

The twentieth century has created a context that overreaches our principles, our ways of being alone and together. Logic fails and the axioms of the old philosophy—the wisdom that we relied on in the past—no longer do justice to our shared worlds. As people and as individuals we have become like sleep-walkers on the edge of a nightmare. We know something is wrong but are not sure if the problem is a dream or a real fact of our lives. And if it is a dream, do we wish to wake to a reality that may be far worse than our imagining? Somewhere and somehow, amidst the boons of technology, the perspective that once guided us no longer serves. We have lost our moral center, the inherent sense of what is right and fair. Answers no longer reflexively follow from the ideals bequeathed us by our past. And yet, the assumptions that supported them are so ingrained in our personal and communal consciousness that it seems impossible to conceive of another perspective that might better serve the present circumstance and the coming millennium.

As problems of principle—of bioethics—each issue is debated by scholars, ethicists, lawyers, pastoral counselors, and most important, the people whose lives are directly involved in medical choices enabled by the extraordinary technologies that have emerged in recent years. When to offer care and when to withhold it, when to deny a request for life support and when to insist upon it: Answers to these now commonplace ethical quandaries elude a resolution acceptable to a range of medical professionals and society in general.

Most of us are divided on these battles. We accept in the abstract arguments about utility but reject in practice their application to those people we know and love. It is one thing to agree with Daniel Callahan that seniors have had "fair innings" and should be denied anything but palliative care.[19] It is quite another to see Mom or Dad or beloved Aunt Janice die for want of specific treatments that might extend their lives. Believing in the principles of individual rights, autonomy, and justice for all, we are unable to apply them in a way that satisfies society as a whole.

Insisting on the absolute definitions of enlightenment philosophy, accepting the assumption of its overriding principles, we find their consistent application difficult when not impossible. Asserting doctrines like those protecting the sanctity of human life, we now have trouble defining the humanness it supposedly protects. Nor can we identify accurately the point where human *life* itself can be said to begin or end. One result has been that the most ardent opponents arguing ethical issues do so from an almost identical set of principles and convictions. And so people of good-will line up on opposite sides of the barricades, insisting their position is the only correct one and that their neighbors, on the other side, are morally corrupt.

The Clash of Absolutes

The result is what Laurence Tribe called a "clash of absolutes," arguments in which fundamental social axioms are accepted equally but interpreted differently by different peoples.[20] Abortion's "pro-choice" advocates insist on the woman's right to control her own body, her own physical destiny. Proponents of fetal rights endorse this principle whole-heartedly—none want to revisit the era when women were defined as male chattel, after all—except when it is used to justify the termination of the not-yet-born in another woman's womb. To them the right of biological self-determination is bounded by those of the "pre-born" because, they insist, that fetus is already a person, a human worthy of the same rights and protections the mother has gained through her membership in society. For their part, pro-choice advocates generally endorse the principle of sanctified human life that "pro-life" advocates argue passionately. But to them the fetus is not yet a living human being and thus falls outside the doctrine's protection.

Both agree on a woman's right to protect her own body; both believe in the sanctity of life. Pro-and antiabortion advocates similarly argue the principles of equality, justice, and self-determination. But one sees only the woman, the mother, the other sees only the fetus, young human life. The result is a paradoxical formulation in which generally accepted statements based on mutually acceptable principles result in distinct and necessarily conflicting conclusions. It is an either/or choice: Either the fetus is a human and thus to be saved, irrespective of the mother, or the woman's right is triumphant, reducing the unborn to biologic irrelevance. As a result, members of every group will take to the streets and to the courts, insisting that their interpretation of what are fundamentally shared ideals is the correct one. And so, among people of principle, there is no room for barter, no allowance for degree; nothing but argument and anger are carried to the streets and to the courts, again and again.

Technology

And so it goes across the landscape of our ethical debates. We are limited by both the perspective of our axioms and by our methods of problem presentation. The result is a series of dilemmas whose urgency grows with each new scientific advance. Who lives, who dies, and who will make that decision? These are questions that will not go away. Many blame these dilemmas on advancing technology and what Margaret A. Somerville calls its "mind-altering knowledge."[21] If only abortion were not so safe and antiseptic then the procedure would be too dangerous to perform and the issue itself would disappear. If only we did not have the power to maintain an anencephalic child, or a PVS (permanent vegetative state) patient, then death would be "natural," and the issue of their maintenance would vanish. Were organ transplantation still just a dream, then its difficult question—who among the equally needy will receive another's vital organ as a rare "gift of life"—would be merely a subject for philosophic speculation. Had we not learned to combat the common killer diseases, there would be so few seniors we would not have to worry about whom to maintain in fragile age. After all, in our grandparents' day there was no class of elderly, only an elite of seniors whose longevity was unusual, rare, and therefore admired.

Others argue that the central issue is not technology's bane but the inadequacy of our methods by which the facts and the context of these dilemmas are first presented and then considered. If our philosophy does not serve—and if nothing else the congress of unresolved bioethical dilemmas is strong evidence it does not—what is needed is not a suspension of medicine's advance but a suspension of the principled approaches with which we address these issues. And so critics of various persuasions have argued in recent years for one or another alternative approach. They range from a "new pragmatism,"[22] to old style, Jesuitical casuistry,[23] from the technologist's "outcome assessment"[24] to the humanist philosopher's discourse ethics. Each has its adherents, but none seem able to achieve a consistent and generally acceptable methodology capable of addressing the complex problems that society must today address.

Whether one blames philosophic methodology or advancing technology, the genie is out of the bottle. It is now clear that an eighteen-century philosophy does not adequately serve a twenty-first century science. As a result, we have principles, and we have issues. On the cusp of the millennium, however, the one does not seem to serve the other. What we need most is what we have yet to consider: a perspective that allows us common ground on which we can discuss together the problems our success has created.

URGENCIES

The problem with principle is not a theologian's dilemma lacking real life heartache and trauma. It is the reality of the daily news, the weekly protest, and the year's Supreme Court calendar. "Moral discourse talk is cases," as Albert R. Jonsen so succinctly put it.[25] From Australia to the Netherlands, time after time, the ethical dilemmas of real persons—of doctors, patients, and patient surrogates—have filled both the news and court calendars for decades: Baby B, Baby C, Baby J, Baby K, Baby M, Baby Doe[26] to Baby Ross,[27] Netty Bootsma, *Buck* v. *Bell*, Nancy Cruzan, *In re T.A.C.P.*, Karen Ann Quinlin, *Roe* v. *Wade*, Sue Rodriguez, Sandra Jensen, Terry Urquart, and Helen Wanglie,[28] to name a few. Each case represents at once the heartache of a single patient and that person's family as well as the soul-testing uncertainty of physicians and nurses involved in disputes over appropriate treatment in the face of physical frailties. Each name on the court calendar—each case recorded in the public record—stands for the scores or hundreds of other patients whose families face similar decisions in anonymity. Beneath the legal and the ethical arguments surrounding abortion, for example, are both the lives of thousands of women who are faced with unwanted pregnancies and those of the now living infants whose mothers may have reluctantly carried them to term. The famous and still controversial U.S. Supreme Court decision, *Roe* v. *Wade*,[29] changed the tenor but did not resolve the core of that debate.

Choices must be made in both the world of law and the realm of medical ethics. What we need is what we do not have: a perspective in the larger sense of the word, a view that makes apparent the sweep of the issues at hand. This lack persists not only because of a clash of personal and societal values, although that is an important factor, but also because we have viewed these issues from a logically constrained eighteenth-century perspective. Either actively or through inherited and institution-alized rules, perhaps more by unconscious default than by intention, society has assumed that the conundrums of modernity have yes-or-no, either/or, right-or-wrong answers. Reliance on this traditional approach, one based on absolute definitions and universal principles, has contrib-uted to the assumption of mutually exclusive categories into only one of which the subjects of our ethical uncertainty must be placed. A patient must be alive or dead, human or nonhuman; a fetus is either a living person or a biologic irrelevance; the abortionist is perceived as either a killer or a blameless, medical technician. Such partitioning of the com-plex human experience into discrete and disjunct categories leads to what Peter Gould called a "tyranny of taxonomy"[30] that inaccurately simplifies complex, multidimensional problems, dichotomizes meaningful nuances, and denies a very human, very real kind of uncertainty.

The result has been a perspective of ethical roulette. It is all red or black, and all chips are down when the dealer spins the wheel. Either we save the fetus or we honor the woman's right to chose. The anencephalic infant is a human being, a person like you or me, or it is a body without a soul; it is a less-than-human nonperson perceived only as a field for transplantable organs. We support seniors or we care for children, focus-ing our health dollars and our expertise on one or the other group. This bivalent, either/or approach based on a priori principle is a legacy of our ancestors, a logical engine that propelled us through the Enlightenment and into the present age. And here, perhaps, is the problem. For reasons this work attempts to make clear, the methodologies of the past are in-capable of resolving the dilemmas we currently face, as individuals and as a society. Indeed, the limits of their arguments have been evident for generations. Simply, arguments from a priori principles using absolute definitions and a yes-or-no, bivalent logic create problems that are insol-uble unless wholly restated.

A RESOURCE PERSPECTIVE

Answers are possible. We can extricate ourselves from the ethical, often paradoxical thickets choking much of medical and medico-legal decision making. This requires neither a wholly new philosophy nor an alternate ethic, but instead an approach that will allow us to see all claimants in a dilemma simultaneously. This book's principal conceit is that tools now used to balance conflicting views over water resources, settlement patterns, and urban development also can be employed in conflicts over appropriate action or nonaction in the arena of medical philosophy and bioethics. Techniques of resource analysis used to balance competing demands for scarce resources offer methodologies by which agreement can be achieved in areas of bioethics where disagreement now reigns.

From the battle over hemodialysis to debates over organ transplantation, we have faced again and again the essential problem of a needy population vying for a limited resource. Indeed, the assumption of at least moderate scarcity has been long assumed to be an essential element of moral conflicts demanding just resolution.[31] Advancing bioethics as an activity self-consciously allocating scarce resources first accepts this context and then seeks a method of both problem definition and conflict resolution applicable to one or another specific concern. What is to be husbanded, however, is not simply a medical or physical resource—hemodialysis machines, transplant organs, hospital beds, and so forth—but the persons whose care is in question. From this perspective the question becomes, first, how do we define our resource base when what is at issue is the life of fragile human beings, and second, what is the best way to act upon those definitions?

Across the range of currently troublesome dilemmas, the goal then becomes to arrive at a solution acceptable to all parties through an approach that will use clearly defined criteria that are demonstrably relevant to a specific bioethical concern. This does not mean ignoring moral principles like equality, justice, or self-determination. Nor does it require a suspension of individual moral judgment and intuition. But because the goal is first and foremost a policy or perspective that is generally acceptable rather than individually satisfactory, principles and perspectives employed must first be defined in a way that can advance a problem solution that can be broadly acceptable to all concerned parties.

This means the first step must be to define an ordering principle, axiom, or intuition focused to the issue at hand ("Who gets scarce organs?"

"What is an appropriate treatment of anencephalics?"). Then the problem is examined in a way that can lead to a generally agreed upon formulation. Thus the perspective advanced here is grounded not in principled argument alone but in an approach that builds from concrete problems to general patterns of resolution. To the extent it is broadly inclusive in its construction, involving a variety of persons concerned with an individual issue, it may more closely resemble a moral anthropology or sociology than a traditional metaphysics.

This approach requires a series of changes in our assumptions about the way in which problems of bioethical and medical uncertainty should be addressed. First, it demands that we view the categories and attributions defining contemporary bioethical decision making as overlapping ranges on a continuum rather than as discrete either/or sets. As the next chapter argues, categories of inclusion or exclusion are rarely clear cut. We also need to understand that cases may belong to more than one category simultaneously. What Stephen G. Post calls "the moral challenge of Alzheimer's disease," for example, is not the sole, exclusive provenance of dementing seniors.[32] The issues of physical and cognitive limits in a progressive disorder are shared by the victims of various categories of disability, including brain tumor and injury. Ultimately, bioethical issues addressing questions of who to treat and how to treat them will affect all those living a restricted life.

Second, there must be a methodology that permits first a systematic analysis, and second, a solution that is generally acceptable to both public and professional communities together. For reasons explained in chapter 3, I have chosen a multicriterion decision-making (MCDM) approach utilizing the Analytic Hierarchy Process (AHP).[33] Multicriterion analysis neither requires nor prohibits absolute answers. It begins, however, with an assumption of complexity permitting partial answers in which the result may be "yes *and* no," rather than either/or. The AHP's use of pairwise comparison of criteria, described more fully in chapter 3, lends itself both to problem definition and a concrete analysis with extensive public input. Finally, both offer mechanisms for broad public participation in the evaluation and decision processes.

This is important because the activity of a resource ethic must be inclusive rather than exclusive. It must involve public as well as professional stake holders in its deliberations. Public concern over bioethical dilemmas—abortion and physician-assisted suicide are two current examples—demonstrate a demand for general as well as professional input. As members of the Seattle "God Committee" learned thirty years ago, no one

group can expect its dictates to be accepted reflexively by all. The days
are gone when jurists, legislators, or ethicists could make a judgment,
hand down a ruling or law and expect the public at large to accept it
without demure. Nor can physicians be expected to serve as the sole or
even the primary arbiters of these dilemmas.

Trained in the concrete and practical, physicians are rarely equipped
for the role of "philosopher kings." Gross anatomy, cellular biology, genetics, histology, and the rest of the modern medical curriculum prepares
the physician to diagnose and treat the physical body, not to adjudicate
philosophical dilemmas or social conflicts. Bioethical dilemmas and the
social issues they simultaneously reflect and define are only secondarily
clinical problems. First and foremost they involve public sensibilities
within a context applying public resources. Thus any approach that attempts to address today's complex of medico-legal dilemmas must permit
real public involvement in its deliberations. As Arthur L. Caplan put it,
"I've come to believe that there is no point in doing bioethics if, ultimately, some of it doesn't take place in public."[34] A multicriterion approach using the AHP has that potential.

Finally, no matter how brilliant the analysis or how logical the suggested remedy, logical brilliance alone will not guarantee resolution to
the dilemmas we face. Practical demonstrations of potential systems of
resolution are necessary. To this end, two "core problems" have been
selected for analysis in chapters 4 through 6. The first concerns who will
be deemed eligible to receive scarce donor organs. How do we choose
between equally needy candidates when all cannot be saved? The issue
of organ donor eligibility is the historical problem of hemodialysis transposed to a new frame. It is also the broader issue of necessary choices
within a context of scarcity and thus of health care rationing.[35] Organ
transplant eligibility problems concretely address the basis on which we
might make a range of decisions affecting socially and physically distinct
persons. While others have argued that organ transplantation allocation
is a model for medical ethics at large—"No part of the health care system
has done more to resolve questions of justice than transplantation"[36] is
the boast—it is used here as a symbol of the limits of modern medical
ethics. If the leaking lifeboat is filled to capacity and beyond, who will
be jettisoned so that the majority might survive?

The second focus problem is the dilemma presented by severely anencephalic infants commonly called "brain stem" babies.[37] The stark
question they present is whether to maintain or let die those with functioning bodies but without higher order cognition. Some suggest what

we decide in this specific context will affect others, including late stage Alzheimer's disease patients and persons in a permanent vegetative state who by reason of injury or illness are both wholly unconscious and unlikely to awake from their comas.[38] More generally, the question is whether or not the traditional doctrine of the sanctity of human life's protective circle should be withdrawn to exclude these cases. Methodologically, the issue is how these determinations can best be made.

It is the specificity of the anencephalic condition—and the attention it has received—that recommends it as a discrete, core problem. While there are degrees of anencephaly, in general it is a relatively rare disorder occurring when a fetus' brain does not develop. The resulting infant is born without a developed brain but with a functioning brain stem permitting autonomic reactions including breathing, grasping, sucking, and so forth. The projected life of such infants is short, and those who survive often need periodic mechanical ventilation, help in breathing. In the cases that have given their name to famous court judgments—*In the Matter of Baby K*,[39] *In re T.A.C.P.*[40]—the question has been whether such an infant is a person like you or me or a nonperson, a less-than-fully–human being who is no more than a collection of body parts to be "harvested" with impunity.

Ultimately, these problems are not just medical or philosophical but also deeply personal and resolutely social. Science can define the developmental failure that creates an anencephalic infant; it can demonstrate the presence or absence of electrical brain function in a comatose patient; it can describe the neurology of progressive paralysis that is the hallmark of Lou Gehrig's disease (amyotrophic lateral sclerosis [ALS]). What it can not do is guide society at large—or its individual members—in determining what these physical states mean. Ultimately, these are all problems of self-definition, of who we will permit within the sanctified boundaries of fully credited humankind. And it is here, where answers are evolving and uncertain, that the activity of resource-based bioethics must focus its abilities.

Because both the issues addressed and the context in which they are presented attempt to define appropriate behavior in complex situations, this work necessarily intrudes upon the domain of both ethics and the philosophic systems that support it. But because its final focus is practical—hospital policies, medical guidelines, and appropriate methodologies to define them—it inevitably encroaches upon issues of politics and political philosophy. As Harvard biologist R. C. Lewontin put it: "Every political philosophy has to begin with a theory of human nature."[41]

Conversely, every theory of human nature will end in a political philosophy. Deciding who is to receive care and who is to be denied, defining and then defending the boundaries of sanctified human life, strikes at the heart of our beliefs about the nature of our species. Thus, while this book attempts to understand our present inability to address certain central problems in bioethics, its conclusions will of necessity extend beyond single issues or limited policies to the broader discourse of philosophy and political science. After all, our ideological prejudices and intellectual histories shape the very forms of our explanation and our science, in the end defining the actions that result from them. And in the search for a new approach to these ethical dilemmas, those patterns of thought and examination provide the critical background for this analysis.

LIMITS

The goal of this work is not the justification or critique of one or another a priori principle. It does not offer the enunciation of a single, definitive answer to either bioethics in general or to a specific bioethical problem. Its interest is first and foremost methodological: By what means do we choose between the needy and the fragile? How can a debate over hard choices best be enjoined, and at what scale of discourse can agreement on these problems be researched? Answers may be acceptable in a community—be it a regional hospital or a nation-state—to the extent that all persons involved in decision making accept its tenants and the results of its application. But they also may be bounded by the assumptions of that community and its culture. Despite the talk of a global community we remain a loose confederation of distinct cultures with values and perspectives that differ widely not only from country to country, but sometimes, from region to region, or community to community.

Limited answers based on local perspectives may be the best that we can honestly present if we hope for agreement, let alone consensus. To achieve a broadly persuasive position it may be necessary to work from the local to a regional or national context rather than to assume a universal principle will easily offer a broad, generally applicable solution. The challenge thus becomes one of assuring the widest possible agreement on a pertinent definition or assumption at a specific geographic scale. The question then becomes not whether answers can be found, but to whom will those answers be sufficient? The real goal of this approach is to seek the axioms and values that have greatest proven demonstrable efficacy and then to apply them at a scale at which their applicability can be demonstrated.

One of the lessons of this analysis—and of the broad history of the boundary between medical and social history—is that no answer will necessarily be true for all people and for all eternity. The days when we could assume that simple axioms reflected self-evident, absolute principles and resultant values is gone. All principles are interpreted and reinterpreted by each generation. There are no iron-clad verities, only query and response in an evolving society. Partial answers to complex, ethical questions is the best that can be achieved. As the next chapter seeks to demonstrate, just as no principle is obvious and absolute, no answer will necessarily serve all nations, or even all medical sites within a single nation.

Of necessity, therefore, answers to our current dilemmas will not be found by reflexive recourse to the works of Immanuel Kant or the writings of other, old-style philosophers who assumed the applicability of absolute principle to a constant world. This is not to say, however, that the insights of the past must be wholly rejected. It may be, in fact, that what results from this activity is a better understanding of the uses that are now being made of older principles, approaches, and axioms. Ideas and ideals like autonomy, humanness, and moral obligation may be maintained but will of necessity be redefined as limited constructs. They can however no longer be assumed to offer clear, unequivocal direction. One can argue that a lesson of our bioethical debates is that Jürgen Habermas was correct when he insisted that ethical norms are not defined by reference to a priori principle and antecedent theory in a form of ethical, spontaneous generation, but instead emerge from a discourse that is only as universal as its acceptance by a community or a group of persons.[42] The questions addressed by the substantive chapters of this book are: How can this discourse be framed, how can it be analyzed, and what is to be learned from framing a community's discussion from the perspective of resource rather than principle?

2

Does the Sanctity of Human Life Doctrine Sanctify Humanness or Life?

In the early 1950s, a violent epidemic of bulbar poliomyelitis swept the industrialized world. Tens of thousands of persons, mostly children, were infected with a virus whose disease course ended, for most, in death from respiratory paralysis. The fortunate few who survived the illness often did so with long-term disabilities. When it was reported that positive pressure ventilation could save many patients, hospitals in Canada, North America, and Europe strained their resources to provide treatment. First-year medical students were pressed into service at many hospitals. They were taught to manually maintain those patients whose respiratory muscles had been permanently damaged by the illness. Eight hours on and eight hours off, they physically kept alive those who otherwise would have died from the disease.

The salvation of a population of thousands of persons whose lives would be spent encased from chin to feet in an "iron lung" requiring long-term supervision and physical assistance was viewed with pride by both the medical profession and by society at large. Saving poliomyelitis patients was saving human life, the physician's first goal. A physically restricted life spent in a breathing apparatus was perceived by all as far better than no life at all. For the medical community it was an at least partial victory over a disease that had been inexorable. For the public at large, it was a triumph of modern medicine celebrated popularly in newspapers and magazines. During the 1960s, *Reader's Digest* would report on patients in the iron lung who became bridge masters, received academic degrees, and otherwise fulfilled life goals despite their physical limits.

By the 1990s, however, medical triumphs at the expense of physical mobility were broadly perceived as social failures. Patients with Lou Gehrig's disease, also known as amyotrophic lateral sclerosis (ALS), were being encouraged by physicians to refuse ventilation—and thus life on a portable respirator—as "no life at all." As the wife of one patient said of her husband's doctors: "They encouraged me, eight of them surrounding me, to let him die, and let him die 'with dignity.' I said, 'I'll take care of his quality of life, thank you very much. You take care of saving his life.' "[1] Others were simply not informed about the possibility of mechanical ventilation as a life-saving measure.[2] Patients with physically restricting illnesses like ALS who chose euthanasia or assisted suicide rather than a restricted life were generally applauded by the public. Some like Noel David Earley, an MS patient, developed Internet Web pages to proclaim their desire to die for an often admiring, computerized audience.[3] Canadian ALS patient Sue Rodriguez was typically described by national TV newscasters as "plucky" and "courageous" in her unsuccessful Supreme Court petition for the right to assisted suicide and against her "terminal" condition. Those like retired pathologist Jack Kevorkian who perform assisted suicide on the physically restricted came to be viewed by many as folk heroes.

The preservation of fragile life appears to have diminished as a goal for both medicine and society in the period between the last polio epidemic and the last decade of this century. And yet, "If we give up the idea of the sanctity and inviolability of bodily life, then a traditional taboo is broken, a wedge is opened for powerful interests to extinguish the demented, ill, immature, aged, or other vulnerable undesirables who cannot defend themselves."[4] What happened to salvation as a primary virtue, to the social and medical assumption advocating a physically restricted life over no life at all?

SANCTITY OF HUMAN LIFE DOCTRINE

What has changed since the polio epidemic of the early 1950s, some bioethicists say, is that the once iron-clad doctrine defining the sanctity of human life has been eroded. We no longer assume that all human beings should be saved, whatever the limits of their future life. All life is neither sacred nor to be protected. In debates ranging from the care of anencephalic infants to the maintenance of fragile seniors, the question has become: Where are the boundaries of sanctified human life? Who falls within its protected sphere?

This, many say, is a signal change in cultural valuation and thinking. As Australian bioethicist Peter Singer observes, "After ruling our thought and decisions about life and death for nearly 2,000 years, the traditional western ethic has collapsed."[5] Paradoxically, most commentators agree that advancing medical technologies are the reasons for this change. "New realities," are forced upon us, says Margaret A. Somerville, by "this new science and technology, and the mind-altering knowledge it makes available."[6] Thus, a new ethic and bioethics are required by our new science. This is the starting point of many commentators, an "obvious" fact. "There is no doubt," writes Joram Graf Haber, "that the miracles of medical technology have brought up ethical issues not contemplated by us until the very recent past."[7] In other words, things were simpler even two generations ago. Back then, we knew where we stood. Things now murky were crystal clear. For the first time in two millennia, the sanctity of human life doctrine is up for grabs.

It is easy to blame technology for the medical dilemmas we face today, to argue about what James J. Hughes calls a "generative force to medical technology."[8] From the impact of in vitro fertilization on our understanding of early life to the new-found ability to maintain bodies in a permanent vegetative state, technology is the cause of the conundrums of contemporary medical ethics. The generally accepted assumption is that a once firm set of principles and definitions based upon the sanctity of human life is now eroding in the face of a generation's stunning scientific advances in medicine and medical technology.

This somehow comforting if narrow perspective ignores the complex history it seeks to address. Without denying the enormity of changes in modern medical knowledge over the last fifty years, they are neither the sole or even the primary cause of the ethical and bioethical dilemmas we now face. To argue that an eighteenth-century philosophy will not serve a twenty–first–century science indicts the philosophy, not the advancing science. New technologies may, however, highlight the limits of the moral ethic we espouse, providing new contexts in which its values may be shown always to have been limited and thus inadequate.[9] Kurt Bayertz calls this "denaturalizing" what once seemed seamless.[10]

ANTECEDENTS

Despite the general insistence that medical advances have crippled a doctrine that was once firmly advanced, the sanctity of human life doctrine has *never* been inviolate. This core value in our tradition has always been a matter of shifting cultural definitions excluding specific groups (enemies, the fragile, those of other races, people of other tribes, religions, or races, etc.), in specific contexts. Exceptions have always been allowed because for centuries the doctrine has been little more—and never less!—than a culture-bound definition of membership and identity. Were the sanctity of life an absolute imperative, we would of necessity all be pacifists refusing to take another person's life for any reason. If its protection was ever as firm as today's ethicists insist, all Western countries necessarily would in the past have abjured capital punishment.

Instead, doctrinal protection traditionally has been reserved for members of a group who define themselves in opposition to other species members in terms of social, economic, political, and religious values. Its application has always been limited. Even when proclaimed as a universal, it has typically been honored more in the breach than through rigorous observance. Like democracy among the ancient Greeks—who restricted participation to a small elite—the sanctity of human life's protection always has been restricted by ruling groups who reserved full membership in the family of man for their own. Who is included in the doctrine's sacred domain has always been a matter of a degree of exclusion.

The problem is not one of simply interpreting and reinterpreting an abstract but well-understood principle so that it can be applied in one or another specific context. More fundamentally, the general principle is not applicable because its individual parts are not clearly defined in a way that is universally accepted. Thus, before one can consider the doctrine, one must look first at what is meant by humanness and life. Historically, the doctrine's emphasis has been on defining *human* life, assuming that viable life itself was easily identifiable. Life was what survived—the beating heart—no more and no less. Over the last eighty years, however, the definition of viable life itself has become a subject of increasingly independent focus. Over the last fifteen to twenty-five years, that problem has given rise to even narrower definitions based on "quality of life" and "personhood" arguments. Let us briefly begin, first, with questions of *human* life before turning to those involving human *life* and the issues of its quality and qualification. If we cannot clarify what the words of the doctrine mean, today, then much of the ethic and law that are based upon it will be open to question.

Human Life

For centuries, religious and cultural affiliations were critical, distinguishing values separating "real" and "good" humans from those who were seen as near-human or subhuman and therefore valued only as commodities or conscripted labor. Sanctified life was at best a matter of theology and salvation, not of general species membership at all. Further, peoples with different skin pigmentation, different levels of technologic development, and those espousing distinct political allegiances have all been deemed, at one time or another, as outside the doctrine's protection. Examples of the exclusion of near-humans can be found in the chronicles of the Christian crusaders' treatment of non-Christian prisoners; of the harsh exploitation of Latin American peoples by their Spanish conquerors; and in the treatment of Native (North) Americans by nineteenth-century descendants of European settlers.

The history of slavery in the United States presents a case study of the denial of full, doctrinal protection to people on the basis of skin pigmentation and country of ancestral origin. Even where religion was not an issue, blacks were defined in law as living property whose lives were no more sanctified or protected than the lives of other farm animals, like an owner's horse or donkey. They could be bought or sold, beaten or otherwise violated with impunity. In this context it is important to remember that earlier in this century Caucasian physicians in the southern United States almost routinely refused emergency treatment to black citizens presenting in distress at white-only hospitals. The story of jazz singer Bessie Smith's death in September 1937, after being refused treatment at a hospital near Chattanooga, Tennessee, is perhaps the best-known modern example of this.[11]

The relevance of doctrinal exclusion on the basis of social and cultural prejudice has been generally obscured, however, by the degree to which recent bioethical debates have focused not on definitions of full humanness, but on those of human *life*. In the end, however this, too, is a difference of degree and not of kind. Questions of human *life*, and the degree to which it is sanctified or allowed to end, have for several generations at least been an issue of sustained and continued argument.

Eugenics

The nineteenth-century eugenics movement, which gained legal legitimacy in the United States in the 1920s—and in Europe soon after—was an attempt to restrict doctrinal sanctity not merely to those accorded the honor of humanness, but more specifically, to those humans whose lives were generally perceived as socially useful, aesthetically pleasing, and therefore worth living.[12] While the fullest expression of this "scientific" definition of sanctified human life was reached in Germany, it was equally evident in other Western countries where social leaders similarly embraced eugenic programs. Eighty years ago in the United States, for example, Dr. Harry J. Haiselden, a well-known Chicago physician, allowed the death of a number of "defective" infants under his care, publicizing those deaths in the Hearst newspapers.[13] The "doctor death" of his day, Haiselden's active advocacy of eugenics—and of euthanasia—were the touch points of a national debate on the cost, care, and place of the fragile in U.S. society in the second decade of this century.

In the 1920s, the court decision of *Buck* v. *Bell* permitted the forced sterilization of "potential parents of socially inadequate offspring," women who were deemed likely to give birth to antisocial individuals, or individuals who would require state support.[14] Supreme Court Justice Oliver Wendell Holmes wrote, in what Stephen J. Gould calls "one of the most famous and chilling statements of our century": "It is better for all the world if, instead of waiting to execute degenerate offspring for crime, or to let them starve for their imbecility, society can prevent those who are manifestly unfit from continuing their kind."[15] This was eugenics in the name of economics and Darwinian progress.

Thus until overturned forty-eight years later by the still controversial U.S. Supreme Court decision, *Roe* v. *Wade*,[16] the sanctity of human life's doctrinal protection did not extend in the United States to the offspring of "unwed mothers, prostitutes, petty criminals, and children with disciplinary problems."[17] An irony of this history is that, in the 1940s, it was determined that the woman whose sterilization was ordered by *Buck* v. *Bell*, Carrie E. Buck, was not mentally unfit. She was simply poor and uneducated when sterilized by order of Mr. Justice Holmes' Supreme Court.[18] Removal of the sanctity of life protection from her potential offspring was not, in the end, a matter of an insupportable "social cost of degeneracy." It was instead a matter of bad science, class economics, social prejudice, and ignorance transformed into institutionalized sanctions against the poor and uneducated.

It was in the eugenics movement that biologic and social definitions of both humanness and protected life were first clearly joined. Exclusion of the socially undesirable or mentally unfit from the sanctity of human life's protective sphere was in part based on the shifting definition of what was perceived as a supportable life, or at least one deemed socially acceptable. And, in a thoroughly modern manner, these exclusions to a presumably iron-clad doctrine were advanced on the basis of social economics (society could not afford to support imbeciles or condone those with a genetic bias to criminal behavior) and parallel considerations of social worth.

We continue to struggle with the same issues. Do economic arguments justify the exclusion of the needy from the full potential of our care? Are there patients whose condition is such that we need not save them? To whom do we advance the protection of common humanity, and to what extent will the fact of physical life—the "beating heart"—be a guarantee of protection? Are anencephalic infants included, or are they merely organ transplant sources to be harvested with impunity?[19] Does life's protected sanctity extend its doctrinal protection to patients in a permanent vegetative state, to late stage Alzheimer's patients, to the nonworking, superannuated senior?

Clearly, these are not new questions. They have been ferociously considered at least since the 1930s, when Germany's Third Reich first instituted broad eugenic policies redefining the boundaries of sanctified human life. It extended the judgment of Mr. Justice Holmes and the North American eugenics movement to justify and carry out, for example, the euthanasia of both infants born with disabilities and frail or otherwise disabled adults. Eventually, more than five thousand infants were put to death because their lives were deemed potentially untenable and thus their places as citizens and humans deemed to be forfeitable.[20] More generally, redrawing the boundaries of protection offered by the sanctity of human life to include only "healthy" life resulted in the murder of more than seventy thousand "defectives" who while living were dispatched because their fragility denied them the protection of species membership.[21]

As Martin S. Pernick notes, German and American eugenicists maintained close ties through the 1930s. Indeed, "German race hygienicists regarded the United States as a leader in applying eugenic theory to public policy, and they carefully followed American immigration, sterilization, and similar laws."[22] What distinguished the Nazi eugenic program from one then active in North America was, first, its consistency; second, its scale; and finally, its combination of older cultural definitions—exclusion by race or religious preference—with those based on then current medical perspectives. Thus, what was a limited state policy in the United States was wholly and comprehensively endorsed by the Third Reich. But North American arguments for the exclusion of "defectives," the frail, and the socially "unfit" from the sanctity of human life's doctrinal protection were consistently heard and often warmly received in many official quarters.

Modern Variants

Similar arguments are at the heart of many of our contemporary bioethical and biomedical debates. From the "Phil Donahue" show to *Scientific American*, "eugenics is back in fashion," proclaimed the latter in 1993. "The primary reason behind the revival of eugenics is the astonishing successes of biologists in mapping and manipulating the human genome."[23] The suggestion that a pregnancy be terminated because the fetus may mature to become an infant with a cleft palate, or an adult with Huntington's chorea (or familial Alzheimer's disease, breast cancer, obesity, etc.) is no more or less than eugenics revisited. It is a determination that the potential of a life so affected is unworthy and therefore outside the doctrine's protective boundaries.

Definitions of a "worthy" life have masqueraded as "science" for years, however. Stephen J. Gould points out that the Wannsee Protocol that defined the Third Reich's "final solution" did so in the name of humanness, the good of the culture and perhaps the species, and on the basis of the then accepted scientific principle of *Natürliche Auslese*, or Darwinian "natural selection."[24] Arguments based on natural selection and economic necessity assured those in both Europe and North America that the frail life—a patient with multiple sclerosis, an infant with Down syndrome, a senior with Alzheimer's—was defined as no life at all. In the United States, this meant, first and foremost, the criminal and the "imbecile." In Germany, it also included the ailing, Gypsies, and German Jews: groups whose lives were assumed to be so different or so fragile as to be outside the protection afforded by the sanctity of life doctrine.[25] The "who" of human personhood became the "what" of expendable, excluded otherhood.

Human Life

Membership in the category of protected living humans remains problematic, as does the values defining that membership. Were doctrinal protection solely anchored in the issue of biologic viability, the extended debate over whether or not to maintain anencephalic infants would be immediately silenced. Paul A. Byrne, Joseph C. Evers, and Richard Niles are clearly correct when they argue that: "When he/she has a beating heart, a measurable blood pressure, some movement, and many functioning internal organs and systems, that baby is alive."[26] To argue otherwise would be, as Judge Clyde Hilton insisted in the judgment known as *Baby K*, to create a class of disabled persons divested of the protection we offer living citizens and thus of their human rights.[27] And yet, there is a growing consensus that anencephalic infants are by definition outside the protection supposedly afforded to all by the sanctity of human life doctrine.[28] They are from this perspective un-persons who may be perceived as living fields for organ harvesting.

The debate over anencephalic infants endures not because medical criteria are in dispute but because the shifting frame of cultural self-definition rather than undisputed biologic fact remains in a state of disputed flux. Anencephalic infants have become a litmus test for a far greater class of nonresponsive, physically viable, biologically alive adults. That class immediately extends, as others have noted,[29] to patients in a permanent vegetative state, and perhaps those in the later stages of diseases like Alzheimer's, Parkinson's, or MS.[30] In all these arenas, the question is not whether or not sustainable human life is evidenced—in each case it is—but whether or not we wish to acknowledge the affected person's humanity and thus the necessity of protection for individuals whose lives are fragile and tenuous.

Advances in medical science thus have returned us yet again to the same old questions of social priority and cultural allegiance. Who do we acknowledge as a living human person and thus worthy of protection? To what extent will we choose to maintain the more fragile among us? Are, for example, Down syndrome persons equal to all others despite their limitations? If the answer is no, then their lives do not deserve equal doctrinal protection. That was the issue raised in euthanasia cases involving otherwise viable infants with Down syndrome—for example, Baby Ross to Baby Doe[31]—and more recently in the debate over whether or not to accept Down syndrome persons as organ transplant recipients.[32]

Advances in genetic testing may expand the field of this debate, but they do not change them. Just as *Buck* v. *Bell* sought to limit future generations of "imbeciles" and the antisocial by forced sterilization, the question today is whether to permit, encourage, or refuse the eugenic pruning of future generations because an individual family history suggests a greater or lesser probability that offspring may develop a serious illness (Huntington's, familial Alzheimer's, breast cancer, etc.) later in life.[33] A related question is whether expensive medical care should be withheld from the frail elderly because they have outlived their usefulness and are assumed to be an expensive drag on the national economy.[34] Put another way, is superannuation a reason to limit the protection of the sanctity of life doctrine?

Animal Rights

For some, the lessons of this history argue that the sanctity of human life doctrine should not be limited to human beings. Members of other species with whom we share genetic patterns and general social characteristics should be protected, too. The animal rights movement, and especially that branch involving the rights of primates, is thus a logical extension to this debate. After all, we share approximately 97 percent of our genetic pattern with our near cousin, the chimpanzee. "Zenotransplantation," the use of primate or pig internal organs for human beings, is now in the experimental stage. With this intimacy, the argument goes, "human life" becomes a gray area whose boundaries may extend beyond the boundaries of Homo Sapiens.

"Why does species membership make such a difference," Peter Singer asks in *Rethinking Life and Death*, "to the ethics of how we may treat a being?"[35] He argues that in defining the sphere of protection offered by this doctrine, that conformity to the human genome is secondary to the criteria of demonstrable intelligence and social interrelation. Human is as human does, in other words. In his construction, killing an intelligent chimpanzee but preserving a severely anencephalic infant—or perhaps a patient in a permanent coma—makes no sense. The first is aware, demonstrably intelligent, and clearly social. The latter is not. Thus, the former and not the latter, he would argue, is deserving of both membership in our community and the protection it affords us all.

This is a telling point in light of the long human history of the sanctity of life's shifting and uncertain boundaries. Its protection has always been sectarian, including one group but not another on the basis of cultural self-definition and self-interest. And, as the one hundred year history of eugenics has demonstrated, "life" has never been an adequate criterion for either automatic exclusion from or inclusion in our protected community. At the least, Singer's argument forces us to recognize that humanness and personhood are cultural definitions, that "life's" definition and boundaries are values and not buttressed facts open to a single interpretation. The sanctity of human life doctrine is and always has been, in all its parts, a social construction.

Singer's argument has found general favor among the many who insist that we acknowledge the "humanity" of at least higher primates, and perhaps other vertebrates, too. Admirers of Jane Goodall and proponents of the Great Ape Project are perhaps the best-known advocates for the doctrinal inclusion of at least some primate species.[36] Others offer data on the moral[37] or emotional life[38] of a range of species as evidence of their "humanness," opening the door to the potential of an ever more inclusive sphere of protected life, with "human" life being merely a subset of a broader category of humanness defined as a function of emotional, moral, and cognitive properties. The long history of shifting cultural definitions of protected human life and the hundred years of eugenic history both suggest that ever greater inclusion, rather than exclusion, is the pattern history has followed.

Some may argue that suggesting an equivalence between eugenic policies of the 1920s, in the United States, and the 1940s in Germany is unfair.[39] To equate the racist victimization of Native Americans, Afro-Americans, and so forth, with the use of primates as organ donors and laboratory subjects will be preposterous to many. It is important to remember, however, that less than two hundred years ago, human beings with dark skin were legally, ethically, and spiritually defined as, at best, near-humans who could be bought and sold.

No more than sixty years ago the frail and disabled in Germany were dispatched because their life was perceived as at once so tenuous and so different as to be legitimately extinguishable. In the 1970s and 1980s, children with Down syndrome like Baby Doe and Baby Ross were allowed to die. Simply, their lives were defined as not worth living.[40] More recently, as the chapters on organ transplant eligibility make clear, the question has been whether to include or exclude Down syndrome persons as possible recipients. In the United States, from 1924 until 1972, the fact of "life" and its potential was insufficient to guarantee legal protection to a range of persons who today we would define as having social, cultural, physical, or cognitive "challenges." It is therefore not unreasonable to assume that future generations may view our contemporary definitions and debates with the same horror and pity we reserve for ancestors who excluded from their community and its protection races and peoples we now accept as equal.

ALTERNATE CONSTRUCTIONS

Some may argue, with Margaret A. Somerville, that human life is, "sacred in some unique and special sense."[41] The manner in which sacred human life is to be distinguished from all others, however, is increasingly difficult to determine. This has lead some writers and ethicists to sidestep these problems and attempt to redefine the doctrine's individual parts. Thus, many today argue the question isn't one of "life" as a sacrosanct quality, but of a "quality of life" that must be first defined and then protected. Others say it is neither unique humanness nor a specific level of life quality that we must seek to preserve but "personhood," the qualities of the sentient and social individual, which is the real core of our values.

Alas, there is no more surety concerning "quality of life" or "personhood" than there is about who is protected under the doctrine of the sanctity of human life. The substitution of "quality of life" for the protected category of "human life" is only the old confusion transposed into a new key. "Few topics are more contentious in biomedical ethics," writes Stephen G. Post, "than 'quality of life,' fueling as it has at least three decades of philosophical, theological, anthropological, and clinical debate."[42]

The popularity of the term "quality of life" has become a catchphrase used by the public at large to describe restrictions that its members would not want to live with and may fear. And yet, "Quality of life cannot be determined simply by defining the severity of resulting disability."[43] What able-bodied persons perceive as an "obviously" unacceptable quality of life may be quite acceptable to the person who sits in the wheelchair, breathes through a ventilator, or is restricted in any other way. It may not be the life they would choose or the life they sought. But for many whose choice is living a restricted life or dying, the decision to live with fragility has lead to a "quality of life" that is more than acceptable.

"It is as though I have been granted extra days in the here-and-now," writes Brian Dickinson, "in the way airlines bestow frequent-flyer miles."

An ALS patient requiring mechanical ventilation, his almost total paralysis requires that he use a computer and eye-blink communication to communicate. As a newspaper columnist, he has written about his own condition. "My circumstance has allowed me to regard my world in greater detail than before," he says, "As with a camera, my narrowed focus, while it cuts out large swaths of a scene, gives a brightness and clarity to the smaller field of view that I take in."[44] Thus while he appears to be a living exemplar of an insupportable quality of life—one wholly dependent and physically restricted—Dickinson, like many others with extreme physical limits, sees his world as rich and full.

More generally, one study of caregivers for persons who, like Dickinson, use artificial breathing apparatus found they seriously underestimated the life satisfaction of the respirator-dependent people with whom they worked.[45] The study involved persons who had survived polio but who, as a result of that illness, needed continuous ventilator assistance. In a similar vein, while only 18 percent of emergency room personnel believe that life is worth living after a spinal cord injury, 92 percent of people who have actually experienced severe spinal chord injuries think a life so restricted is indeed worth continuing.[46]

We are therefore faced with a curious situation. Professionals and the public argue there is a minimum "quality of life" that should be the base against which standards of care are measured. Those facing unacceptable lives therefore should be offered—and perhaps urged—to forgo treatment and accept "death with dignity." Many of those living supposedly unexpected lives think differently, however, and they are lionized as a result. In 1997, for example, former *Elle Magazine* editor Jean-Dominique Bauby, locked in following a stroke in 1995, published a book about his condition. A person "locked-in" is one who has lost all physical movement and control, one who cannot use hands, legs, or voice. A person in this state can only communicate by eye blinks—if at all. Dictated letter by letter, eye blink by eye blink, his book became an immediate bestseller in France. Praised for its insights into the richness and the frustrations of this level of disability, it has since been translated into English as *The Diving-Bell & the Butterfly*.[47] Bauby, the editor turned writer, became a star.

In the same vein, few people understand the work of physicist and author Stephen Hawking, a man who has lived with ALS for more than twenty years. While the complete paralysis this disease causes has become emblematic of an unacceptable quality of life, the image of Hawking in his wheelchair has become almost as famous as the Karsh portrait of

Albert Einstein, looking sad and wise, sold on posters and postcards around the world. We shudder at the idea of full paraplegia, of losing control of bodily functions, but we praise Christopher Reeve for his equanimity in the face of paralysis. That the actor whose fame stems from his movie role as Superman is himself now wholly paralyzed following a riding accident adds irony and poignancy to his stance. His life is restricted, but in story after story, the strengths of his life on a ventilator and in a wheelchair have become the stuff of popular legend and hope.[48]

And so we praise those who find meaning in a physically restricted life while simultaneously advancing standards that define extreme physical restrictions as representing an unacceptable quality of life. It is for this reason that ALS has become a primary battleground in the euthanasia argument. As of September 1996 the ratio of ALS to cancer patients dying at the hands of Jack Kevorkian was 1:2, a remarkable figure given the ratio of ALS to cancer cases in that year, which was 1:90.[49] Simply put, progressive paralysis and its attendant need for assistance defines for many a restricted life that is not worth living. Dependence places persons so restricted beyond the sanctity of human life's protection. All that is left for them is the facilitation of a fast and painless death.

In the last great North American polio epidemic, vast monies were spent in the attempt to save poliomyelitis victims. In 1952 and 1953, wards were filled with huge, cumbersome iron lungs that encased the patient from the neck down, breathing for those persons whose respiratory muscles were no longer able to do the job. This was a fact of pride in most hospitals and most communities. It was, we believed then, a triumph of technology to save these lives, even if they were saved to a physically restricted life. Persons whose lives were maintained by those clumsy iron lungs continue, today, on portable ventilators. Like us, they live lives of cheerful anonymity and periodic crisis. And yet were today's "quality of life" standards to be taken seriously, those lives would have been defined as unworthy of continuation.

In the same vein, ethicists like Helga Kuhse and Peter Singer have insisted that conditions like Down syndrome "mean a necessarily reduced potential for a life with the unique features which are commonly and reasonably regarded as giving special value to human lives." The conclusion, Kuhse and Singer argue, is that "the possible benefits of successful surgery in the case of a Down's syndrome child are, therefore, in terms of these widely accepted values, less than the possible benefits of similar surgery in a normal child."[50]

But persons with Down syndrome, and the relatives of persons with this condition, argue vehemently that these "widely accepted values" are neither widely held nor acceptable, and they do not measure the rich potential of lives that are ended in their application. It is, these advocates insist, an unacceptable moral judgment based on prejudice, misinformation, and perhaps, on fear of those who are different. "But there is really nothing God-like in such a judgment," argues another respected bioethicist. "It is not a moral judgment we are making if we think that someone's life is so empty and unhappy as to be not worth living."[51] It is hard, however, to think of anything more morally judgmental than to conclude another's life is not worth living, especially on the basis of amorphous and ill-defined definitions of "worthiness" or life quality.

Similarly, one philosopher likened persons with severe dementia to dogs, since they are assumed to "lack capacities for hopes and fears, dreads and longings for their futures."[52] Implicit in this suggestion is the idea that since we "put down" our pets when they are sick, shouldn't we do the same for our ailing loved ones? Advocates for those with dementia would object that patients with Alzheimer's disease do not lose all human emotion and desire until, perhaps, the disease's last stage.[53] Across the long course of this chronic but not rapidly terminal disease, persons slowly lose cognitive abilities until, in the last stages the ability to think or feel may finally be lost. But it is among the heart-breaking facts of the disease that persons with Alzheimer's, while fragile, will for years display a range of loves, hopes, and emotions that are more poignant for being lost, to them, in a disorder of memory.

Attempts by ethicists and philosophers to separate "acceptable" from "unacceptable" qualities of life on the basis of physical fragility or "mental competence" are reminiscent of the perception and language of the international eugenics movement earlier in this century. In 1920, for example, Dr. Karl Binding and Dr. Alfred Hoche published a monograph entitled *Permitting the Destruction of Unworthy Life: Its Extent and Form.* In it, Binding wrote, "I find no grounds—legally, socially, ethically, or religiously—for not permitting the killing of these people, who are the fearsome counter image of true humanity, and who arouse horror in nearly everyone who meets them." This group included, "incurable idiots, no matter whether they are so congenitally or have (like paralytics) become so in the final stage of suffering . . . their life is completely without purpose, but they do not experience it as unbearable. They are a fearfully heavy burden both for their families and for society."[54] In a thoroughly modern fashion, Hoche argued that even if restricted lives could be shown to be emotionally rich and socially related, maintaining them would be economically counterproductive.

Increasingly, cost is again being used as a determinant in defining health care procedures. Hastings Center's ethicist Daniel Callahan, for example, has argued that economic constraints will require us to withdraw care from some fragile populations if we are to maximize the lives of other citizens. Unlike Justice Holmes in *Buck* v. *Bell*, however, it is not idiots and degenerates but seniors whose maintenance, Callahan argues, is too costly and without sufficient return. They no longer serve—they've had their day—and thus should accept diminished care.[55] This argument can be easily extended to all those who are fragile, restricted, and living short-ened life spans. In this interpretation, the sanctity of human life is re-defined as the sanctity of socially useful human life, or perhaps, as the cost efficient human life. The problem remains. What some see as "un-acceptable" others may see as required. Who decides and on what basis?

Personhood

Another attempt to rewrite the sanctity of human life doctrine has focused on the issue of "personhood." From this perspective it is not humanity itself that we seek to sanctify and preserve, but the human person in his or her complexity. The argument is that the sanctity of human life was never designed to protect all human beings, only those whose characteristics give them, in James W. Walter's words, "a morally unique claim to existence."[56] The essential claim of personhood propo-nents is that sanctity is defined not by the beating heart or the warm body, but by "capacities for significant cerebral functioning." As John Harris put it, "it is only to persons, that is, those individuals who have the capacity to value their existence that respect is owed."[57]

A huge literature has grown around the idea of personhood, especially personhood defined by cognition. Some of this material will be reviewed in a later chapter but, in general, most would agree with Loyola Univer-sity's Dave Thomasma that, "Personhood includes, as essential compo-nents, consciousness, the ability to communicate, and self-awareness."[58] Consciousness, he then explains, means being self-conscious, aware of the world as organized by one's perceptions, of one's body and the physical world, and of mortality itself.

This standard would exclude not only the patient in a permanent coma and the anencephalic infant, but *all* infants at the time of birth. Thus, by a standard of personhood, depending on cognition, infanticide would be permissible, and until they could display the characteristics of self-awareness and self-consciousness, infants would be disposable. To close this gap, most agree that "personhood" is also conveyed on those with the potential to achieve whatever characteristics the definition requires. "Potentiality," James W. Walters tells us, "means the infant's projected capacity to approximate a mature person's mental and physical condition."[59] Think of the normal infant, then, as a "pre-person" and the patient in a permanent coma as, perhaps, a "post-person."

Who defines these conditions, however? What do distinctions like pre-person and post-person mean to the world of treatment and in our ethical world? Are they sufficient for life and death decision making? As animal rights activists make clear, many primates appear to fulfill all the characteristics of personhood—they have speech, are self-conscious, and demonstrate intelligence—although they are clearly neither human, in the traditional sense, nor included in traditional definitions of personhood.

Many would argue that personhood (and thus doctrinal protection) ends with the onset of a persistent vegetative state, that life in a permanent coma is "no life at all." Even that is rejected, however, by those who live with and care for such patients. Stephen G. Post quotes a 1993 story from the *Cleveland Plain Dealer*, for example, describing a husband whose wife was in a persistent vegetative state for many years. She was on artificial feeding and sometimes required mechanical ventilation to breathe. And yet, during football season he would wheel her into the nursing home's common room on Sundays to watch the Cleveland Browns football games together on TV. They both wore the jersey of their favorite quarterback in honor of their local team.

"This story indicated that for some people," Post commented, "even the PVS condition does not disqualify a loved one from equal moral standing under the principle of do no harm. It further suggests that the concept of quality of life might be the quality of lives, including family members."[60] Thus, the very notion of the independent life, of decisions based on the single person's condition, judgment, or perceptions is brought into question. It is not always a question of whether life exists in a human person, Post suggests, but the relation of that beating heart to another's.

Here no less than in the realm of life quality, in other words, the boundaries of human life remain shifting and uncertain. Oliver Sacks, the self-styled *Anthropologist from Mars*, presents case after case of persons with neurological problems that challenge existing definitions of personhood. In one, a patient with Korsakov's syndrome has lost the ability to process new data. "He is, as it were, isolated in a single moment of being," Sacks notes, "with a moat or lacuna of forgetting all around him. . . . He is a man without a past (or future) stuck in a constantly changing, meaningless moment."[61] His memory is stopped in 1945, and new data can only be held for the briefest moment in his memory. The condition of his illness has extinguished a clear self-awareness or self-consciousness in the present day, conditions necessary for personhood, according to many bioethicists. In addition, he lacks a functional sense of time, of the relation between the future and the past without which, others insist, personhood cannot be acknowledged. And yet, to anyone meeting him, Sacks reports, he is indisputably a person and exquisitely, poignantly human; a pleasant and engaging man able to talk about the world he lives in, albeit one whose boundaries are far different from ours.

In perhaps his most famous work, *Awakenings*, Sacks describes his work with a group of patients who had survived the encephalitis epidemic of the 1920s, albeit in a catatonic state.[62] All were maintained in an institution for more than forty years until, in 1969, Sacks treated them with medication that had served to assist Parkinson patients—L-dopa. The patients "awoke" under the effect of the drug, Rip Van Winkles who had slept through the Great Depression and World War II, came back to consciousness expecting to see their young children who had in the interim, become adults. Gradually, however, the effects of the drug began to wear thin, and some patients returned to a catatonic state. The miracle drug was, in the end, only partially effective.

For the thirty years of their near total clinical isolation, Sacks' patients would not have qualified as "persons," as sentient and self-aware individuals. They thus would have failed the standard of "personhood" under any set of criteria advanced by contemporary bioethicists. Were they self-aware and autonomous human beings active in their environments? Certainly not. They were nonaware, nonconscious, physical bodies. During the period of their awakening, they were clearly persons, however: human beings able to think, feel, and perceive in ordinary ways within what was an extraordinary context. And then, some returned to their former, suspended state. Again in suspension awaiting a new treatment and another chance, did they become again nonpersons, human bodies but not human beings to whom we owe allegiance?

In the same vein, it is obvious that their "quality of life" during the catatonic phase was not only not acceptable but in fact nonexistent. Had modern advance directives been popular when those patients were first hospitalized, Sacks' patients would almost surely have been allowed to die, with the method of their death depending on the wording of the directive they completed in wellness. They were maintained, however, because until recently the idea of letting such a person starve to death, or killing them because of physical and cognitive restrictions, was generally perceived as insupportable. Even though there was no hope for a cure or of substantial improvement in their conditions, no "quality of life" and no indications of "personhood," the sanctity of human life doctrine demanded their maintenance. And so we praise the fragile triumph of their awakening through the introduction of L-dopa while attempting to assure, through modern ethics, that in the future patients like them will not need to endure—and we will not be required to fund—the indignity of a wholly restricted, largely unaware institutionalized life.

HUMANNESS AND LIFE

Clearly, new formulations have not solved the conundrum of the sanctity of human life doctrine's applications. If anything, they have drawn traditional debates into greater, bolder relief. The clinical context is not at issue, our social response to fragility is. The birth of a child with Down syndrome, or anencephaly, is an observable fact. So, too, is a diagnosis of bulbar poliomyelitis, Korsakov's syndrome with complete retrograde amnesia, dementia, or ALS. What is in question is the degree to which these and other deficits will include a social diagnosis removing the afflicted person from the protection we offer all members of our community. In the end, what is at stake is not merely how we perceive the fragile among us—or our biological cousins—but how we define ourselves. This is a question reaching beyond medicine and science into politics or at least political philosophy. At issue are not questions of health and disease, of cost and benefit, but of how we wish to define ourselves as a culture and as a species.

We can, should we choose, answer questions of species self-definition and allegiance on the basis of cost effectiveness, saving only those whose continued life may serve our economy, dispatching those nonpersons who seem useless. As theists believing in the divine creation, we can decide that whatever its state that all human life—beginning at the moment of conception—is valuable and thus that no life that can be saved should ever be extinguished. As anthropologists and historians and philosophers, we can comb the literature and seek, in the accumulated data of societies at large, new answers to these old issues.

Any or all of these are defensible positions. But which should govern our policy and the realities of daily treatment? Old approaches have not been able to resolve these issues, and after all these years, it is unlikely their champions in bioethics can forge agreement on such fundamental questions. The problem with principle and its applications will not be resolved by minor changes in our organizational structure—employing bioethicists to assist medical personnel in making critical decisions—or through a complex of progressively narrower, more limiting definitions. Substituting quality of life for human life, or personhood for humanhood, will not resolve our ethical debates. Such responses do not answer the structural, deep-rooted failure of our approach to these dilemmas.

The next chapter argues that an obstacle to resolving these uncertainties is the logic and the approach we have so far used to analyze them. This is not because we have been less than astute, but because the approach itself is limited. Thus, any future resolution marrying our ethics to our medicine, one whose definitions stand a chance of general acceptance, must employ a radically different approach.

3

The Devil's Details: The Limits
of Principle?

Our inability to find generally acceptable social solutions to the dilemmas of modern bioethics results from the way we formulate the rules and principles by which we currently address complex moral issues. For reasons this chapter attempts to make clear, argument from principle alone can never be more than a very general guide to the resolution of specific bioethical problems. While they may serve to express elements of an individual's moral intuition or prejudice they cannot resolve questions of social policy or clinical choice in areas of medical uncertainty. This is equally true of first order principles like the sanctity of human life doctrine, midlevel principles that derive from them, and the resulting axioms of rights and obligations we reflexively use to apply those axioms to our world.

Moral principles are definitions, statements of general, often ill-defined values important to a society and culture at a specific time. They are also abstractions. As such, in any instance their potential as engines of broad, communal resolution is of necessity quite limited because, "Abstraction purchases agreement on principles at the price of disagreement about their interpretation."[1] But it is only through clear definition and interpretation that they can be practically applied. Thus, the supposedly constant sanctity of human life doctrine, to take one example, could be variously interpreted to include or exclude almost any group of fragile persons and members of various races and species.

To be useful, interpretation depends on both clear, precise definitions and a means to apply them to a specific problem. Abstractions by definition lack that specificity, and reasoning from principle lacks a system of focused application. One may say, as John Rawls does in a discussion of fair equality of opportunity, that "these matters are nearly always open to wide differences of reasonable opinion," and that they stem from "complicated inferences and intuitive judgments that require us to assess complex social and economic information about topics poorly understood."[2] If a principle does not serve to narrow the range of opinion, however, to focus intuitive judgments in complex situations, then it will not contribute to the resolution of the challenges presented at the interface of medicine and society. The result will be no more than a value statement without a real world referent, a broad, idealized principle whose meaning is disassociated from any context permitting specific application. Separating principled statement from detailed interpretation leaves only a broad moral intuition that cannot serve as a guide to the formulation of a generally acceptable policy solution in an area of social conflict or medical uncertainty.

The traditional view has been that while moral principles may be clear, that their application to complex issues is by definition "essentially contestable." Disagreement is the inevitable result of judging complex reality through the lens of principled vision.[3] This is necessarily true, however, only if one assumes one must move from abstract principle to practical dilemma. I am arguing that knowing is at the least a two-way street. An ascent from the concreteness of real problem analysis may be, in the end, a principle that is not abstract and essentially contestable but one formulated in a manner that is contextually rich and at least potentially useful.

The devil is in the details. To be applicable, principles must be composed of specific criteria, words or phrases (sanctity, human, life) that are clearly defined, generally understood, and clearly applicable to a context or problem. Second, there must be a means by which the resultant criteria can be applied to a problem. Without the latter, the relation between even well-defined principle and a specific, clinically based problem will be at best, problematic. Until and unless its parts are clearly formulated in a context that offers at least the promise of problem definition and resolution, a principle is simply a sentiment without practical application, a value unto itself.

This reverses our traditional order of knowing. It means that well-defined and applicable principle is not the instrument that allows us to resolve a problem but is, instead, the end result of a problem's resolution. The real issue is not the applicability of the sanctity of human life doctrine, but the definition of its parts. Defining its parts—or those of any principle—therefore must be a goal of bioethics rather than a centerpiece of its approach. The first part of this chapter explains why reflexive argument from principle has not and will not answer the challenges medical ethicists and society must face together. This chapter's latter section describes a methodology for criteria definition and application. Because this is not a philosophic tract but one whose aim is to find a means of better addressing specific bioethical concerns, these arguments necessarily will be sketched rather than argued exhaustively. The intent is first to identify and then avoid the traps that currently frustrate attempts to find practical answers to the complex questions of bioethics.

If this task is to be successful, principled criteria must be defined and then applied in a manner that does not result in either/or, yes-or-no answers to complex problems. It must permit gradations and shadings along a responsive continuum. One result of the traditional, principled approach has been to create a perspective in which only two possible, opposing choices were presented as possible. As Timothy E. Quill and Gerrit Kimsma recently put it in a discussion of euthanasia that might apply equally to a broad range of contemporary biomedical debates: "Individuals are forced to choose between being 'pro choice' or 'pro life,' while most want policies to both favor life and allow choice. [But] public debates tend to be win-lose and either-or, giving a disproportionately loud voice to political extremes."[4]

Across the field of our ethical concerns, a win-lose, either/or choice is simply too limited. It does not reflect the clinical or the social gradations inherent in the problems we face today. The result is a frustrating, logical two-step that transforms ethical problems into what, to the average person, appears to be unsolvable, ethical paradoxes. What is required, however, is an approach that presents at least the possibility of gradated solutions that can open bioethics and the perspective it advances to more open and realistic solutions.

SORITES PARADOX

Given that moral principles are abstractions without clear definition or context, contemporary arguments from principle take on the flavor of a Sorites Paradox. These are problems of membership and definition consisting of, "categorical propositions that can be represented as (or decomposed into) a sequence of categorical syllogisms such that the conclusion of each syllogism except the last one in the sequence is the premise of the next syllogism in the sequence."[5] Zeno called this the problem of the heap. Consider a pile of sand on the beach. If you remove a single grain is it still a sand heap, he asked. Remove another grain and ask again. If one has the time and patience, the process can go on until the entire heap is scattered across the beach. At any point where one says "Stop, it is no longer a heap," and the question is asked, "Why this grain and not the previous one, or one more grain?"

If A, then B; if B, then C . . . if Y, then Z. No choice is obviously better than the other. At each point, another answer is demanded. Every choice, in the end, is an arbitrary judgment. Aristotle explained the problem nicely when he asked: If one plucks out one hair from a man with a full head of hair, is he then bald? If another is plucked out, is the head then bald? At what point does the change from covered to bald occur? There is, however, no single point where the evidence allows a clear distinction between "bald" and "hirsute." There is in Aristotle's formulation no way to say, "I'm balding, which means I'm hirsute on the sides and bald on top." It is always either/or, one or the other. Both states do not exist simultaneously. Sorites-style paradoxes demand absolute categories in contexts where partial membership between categories is required if a reasonable answer is to be formulated. Denying process, it prohibits inclusive answers.

Many of our more difficult contemporary bioethical dilemmas have the flavor and appearance of a Sorites-style formulation. The unending debate over abortion, for example, rests for many upon defining the moment a fetus becomes a human being, the instant we come into existence. When a being is recognized as a living human, as a member of the species, he or she is imbued with the full packet of rights we assign to all members of our species, rights that society must protect. The second before, it is outside the protection the sanctity of human life doctrine accords us all. Along the continuum of humanness, does human life begin three seconds, three minutes, or three months after conception? Does humanity and its subset, personhood, start at the moment of physical birth, or as Orthodox Jewish law insists, thirty days after an infant's first lusty cry? Roman Catholicism asserts that sanctified human life begins with the act of insemination itself. Scientists addressing the issue variously describe our beginning as occurring at the moment of conception; when pulse and respiration are first evident;[6] with the first evidence of synaptic electrical activity in the fetus' eighth week;[7] when more constant, synaptic activity is evident (twenty weeks);[8] or after perhaps thirty-two weeks of development when sustained synaptic pattern is evident.[9] It can as easily be defined as occurring at the moment when the fetus can first exist independently but with medical assistance or at the moment of natural birth.

All answers are right because all are ultimately arbitrary choices along a Sorites-like continuum. Each depends on interpretation of the qualities that are the basis for our self-definition. Answers can be grouped around definitions of human life as a process of cellular development or in terms of synaptic and then cerebral activity. Each specific answer can be contested, each leads to a prior position along the continuum of existence. If synaptic activity is what we mean by human life, then why must it be sustained activity or even frequent? If it is independence that defines us, at what stage do we recognize its presence? And if the key is the process of cellular development, why should it be when the human shape is recognizable? Why not earlier, when mitosis begins, defining the genetic principle of the independent being who will, if there is no crisis, eventually emerge and develop? However one defines the problem, there is a sliding scale of reality that leads inexorably from one conclusion back to its predecessor.

The problem is inverted in debates over "futility" and end-of-life decision making. The question then becomes not the exact moment when life begins, the instant of induction into humanity, but the precise point of human life's cessation. Does it end when self-awareness ceases, even if the body continues? Do we choose a "whole brain" definition, which would grant the status of continuing human life to patients with brain stem but not cortical function, or a "high brain" definition that defines death as cessation of cortical function?[10] Are physicians who maintain patients with "persistent brain death"—the aggressive maintenance of bodily function despite the continued cessation of brain and brain stem functions—attending to living patients or playing with corpses?[11] Indeed, are these even the correct questions? Paul A. Byrne and Richard G. Niles argue that we should reverse the usual orientation and search not for signs of brain death but of brain life lest we pronounce dead a living, breathing human being.[12]

No wonder that ethicists, finding agreement on these definitions impossible, have substituted more limited if not more serviceable constructs for the sanctity of human life's broad doctrinal nouns. But this simply transposes the problem to another line, one in which the problem itself is retained. What are the qualities that make human life worth living? If they include physical autonomy and independence, do we therefore insist that the lives of physicist Stephen Hawking, whose Lou Gehrig's disease has made him technology dependent, and actor Christopher Reeve, wholly paralyzed and largely ventilator dependent since a high spinal injury, are untenable? Do we accept or deny the personhood of a physically independent but perhaps mentally restricted person with Down syndrome? What about the poststroke, aphasic senior who while aware is unable to speak or walk without assistance? Abstract principle offers a plethora of potential interpretations without a method to judge between or then apply them.

Anencephaly

The debate over anencephaly demonstrates how a Sorites-style formulation prohibits the statement of a consistent, principled response to a problem that is at once clinical, legal, and social. Is a severely anencephalic infant—one born with a functioning brain stem but without cortical awareness—a live human being, a person, or simply a body without consciousness, a nonperson whose almost humanity disqualifies it from full care and treatment? If that infant is a living human person then he or she must be cared for to the extent we value and protect human life. If it is a nonperson, a less-than-human being, then its continuance is of no consequence. Except by divine revelation, how can the point of being be precisely defined on the continuum of humanness?

In one well-known case concerning an anencephalic infant, Teresa Ann Campo Pearson,[13] the court ruled that the infant—lacking cerebral but possessing brain stem function—should be kept alive because there exists no single, widely accepted definition of a point along the continuum of humanness at which those who are accepted as human beings can be distinguished from those who are to be excluded. In the absence of a clear and generally accepted definition of when a physically viable life is to be deemed unworthy, the Florida Supreme Court ruled that the law must err on the side of the support of human life no matter how tenuous or fragile. To do otherwise would be to create a class of human nonpersons whose rights were arbitrarily suspended and whose worth was diminished.

At one level, the question is: What are the qualities of human life and who—or what—demonstrates those qualities? Where those qualities lie defines the state's "life interest" in upholding the sanctity of human life doctrine and protecting it for all within its jurisdiction. In cases like this, however, the argument often focused at the level of human person or what Ronald Dworkin calls "constitutional personhood." Is the anencephalic infant in question a living person under the law, and thus to be protected by the state's "life interest," or is it somehow a legal nonperson and thus unprotected?

This was the question addressed in the well-known and still controversial *Baby K* decision. Is an anencephalic infant without cognitive ability or the potential for mental development a person equal to all others? If an anencephalic child is a human person under the law, then the complex of principles mandating care for us all must be applied to it. If it is a nonperson, however, then no care need be given. In 1993, Virginia District Court Judge Clyde Hilton ordered a hospital to continue stabilizing life support for a severely anencephalic infant who needed periodic ventilation if it was to be kept alive. Judge Hilton ruled that in law the anencephalic Baby K was an individual like all others and therefore deserving the same protection as any individual from the law.[14] There was, he concluded no reason to assume the infant's lack of cerebral function, need for medical assistance, or poor life expectancy (under eighteen months) placed it in a class of nonindividuals, nonpersons outside the protection of our justice tradition. Even so disadvantaged a child, Judge Hilton wrote, is no different in law from an AIDS patient with an unfavorable long-term prognosis, is no less deserving of treatment than patients with other serious illnesses. It therefore has society's full protection.

While logically and legally consistent, this judgment seems experientially inappropriate. As friends and neighbors of people living with HIV-complex symptoms, or with those of any life threatening disease, we know intuitively that there is a difference between a person who lives among us with a serious illness/disease and a severely anencephalic infant born with only minimal, autonomous brain stem level functions. The neighbor who plays the organ in the neighborhood church, the woman who gives candy to our children on Halloween, who brought over a dinner when we were ill, is qualitatively different to us from the infant maintained on a respirator who will never share our love, never fulfill our hopes, will never respond to our actions toward it.

This is moral intuition, a feeling that the definitions of the law do not reflect the prejudices of our lives. The difference we perceive between the anencephalic and the AIDS-infected neighbor is manifest. Along the continuum of humanness and personhood should be, we think, a dividing line in which the lives of our sentient neighbors is recognized above those of infants who breath but do not perceive. What this means in terms of the range of care that must be provided to either is not clear, however. If one wants to translate that intuition into a hospital policy that will avoid court censure—one comprehensible to and accepted by a broad community—moral intuition is not enough. What is required is what we do not have, a system allowing both the anencephalic infant and the AIDS-infected adult to be seen as different and equal, simultaneously.

MIDLEVEL PRINCIPLES

The sanctity of human life doctrine is a first-order principle from which midlevel corollaries may be derived. These include equality, because if we value life in general then we value equally its presence in all parties; justice, because we do not distinguish between the value of different human lives; self-determination and autonomy because they are qualities we perceive as important to the state of "personhood," and perhaps humanness itself.

The general paradigm of bioethics is based on deductive reasoning from a limited set of these middle-level principles that ethicists attempt to apply to specific problems.[15] "Biomedical moral problems can be analyzed in terms of four basic moral principles or values that almost everyone, on reflection, accepts as being prima facie valid—along with reflection about the scope of application of each of these principles."[16] They include:

- Autonomy and self-determination, qualities to be valued and nurtured in every human being
- Nonmalfeasance, or the obligation to do no harm
- Beneficence: maximizing benefits and minimizing harms
- Justice and equality: fairness in the distribution of both benefits and burdens among all members of the population.[17]

These are prima facie values principled abstractions. As such they are still ideals without referents and therefore equally open to diverse interpretation.[18] Is it justice, for example, to deny organ transplant eligibility to persons with Down syndrome? Is it doing no harm to allow a hydrocephalic infant to die, thus saving it from an unacceptable "quality of life"? It depends on how one first defines and then applies the principles of justice or nonmalfeasance and what one means by "quality of life." As abstractions, the applicability of these principles is never clear. Even were they somehow resolved so there was no question about their meaning and potential use, still a more fundamental problem would remain. If we are not sure who is and who is not a protected human being—if the applicability of the sanctity of life doctrine itself is uncertain—then we will never be sure who to include among the class of persons to be equitably treated and beneficently considered. If the person with Down syndrome and the hydrocephalic are human beings like you and me, persons under the law, then disallowing their care would seem to be unjust, discriminatory, and a violation of the values and the principles we espouse.

Rights

This is why arguments based on individual rights necessarily fail to answer complex questions like abortion, euthanasia, and the level of treatment appropriate to fragile persons. "Affirmation of basic rights spring from a commitment to the value of the [living human] individual," Loren E. Lomasky says in *Persons, Rights, and the Moral Community*. "From this all else follows."[19] If we value ourselves, our species, then our commitment to the whole must include the persons who are its individual parts. The primacy of the individual, a representative of the whole is, as John Rawls says in A *Theory of Justice*, the "first principle" of our justice tradition, the foundation of our rules of law and government.[20] From it follows the corollary of equality, that no distinction be made between individuals who by definition are equally vested with an identical packet of legal, moral, and social rights.[21]

But if we cannot define what we mean by humanness in general then it is unclear who we will value and protect as an individual representative of the species. Asking whether anencephalics have a right to care depends on whether one thinks they have at least constitutional personhood. Ultimately, that will depend in great part on whether they are seen as qualifying as living human beings. At each stage—humanness, life, personhood—there is a continuum along which one ranges from "yes, of course" to "nope, no way." Analysis leads backward, as it did when life begins or ends. There is no way to clearly choose an answer that everyone will accept. And because the principles upon which resultant rights all rest are abstractions purchased at the price of precise and applicable definition, the "first principle" is one whose subject will always be unclear.

Thus, there is the long debate over whether the focus of ethical debate should be the discrete individual at all. Charles Taylor argues in *The Ethics of Authenticity*, for example, that we are individuals only to the extent that we are social beings.[22] The commitment to the individual is to a discrete person without a social context. Humanness and personhood can as easily be seen as communal definitions. Oliver Sacks put it well when he insisted, in *Awakenings*, that, "Reality is given to us by the reality of people."[23] If individuality resides first and foremost in the social sphere, then individual rights are rooted in the social context. It is something we give or withhold by our communal actions rather than a self-evident quality bred into the bone and born of a unique distinction present in us all, whoever "we" are.

IRRESOLVABLE CONFLICTS

Even were problems of definition resolved, there is still the problem of choosing between two or more apparently conflicting principles or their resulting rights. One cannot conclusively argue that "my rights are more important than yours," any more than one can insist that "this right is more important than that one." Just as all individuals are assumed to be equal, so too are all rights and principles supposed to be equally true. But bioethical dilemmas demand that choices be made within a specific context, and this may mean that apparently equal rights or individuals must be prioritized, with one taking precedence over another. Principled argument provides no mechanism by which this can be done easily, however. The result has been a paradoxical conflict pitting supposedly equal rights—or rights-based claims—against each other.

Abortion provides a convenient example of what this means. Pro-abortion proponents insist that the individual woman's right to biological self-determination and autonomy allow them to unilaterally abort a fetus. Antiabortion activists do not dismiss the woman's right to biological self-determination. They do insist, however, that the fetus is a human being whose right to life must be protected. If these two rights are in conflict, they insist, the right to life must be upheld. What results is, in the words of Lawrence Tribe, a "clash of absolutes" in which choices are absolute, limited, and necessarily opposing.

> In much of the debate over abortion in our society, one side or the other is reduced to ghostly anonymity. Many who can readily envision the concrete humanity of a fetus, who hold its picture high and weep, barely see the woman who carries it and her human plight. To them, she becomes an all but invisible abstraction. Many

others, who can readily envision the woman and her body, who cry out for her right to control her destiny, barely envision the fetus within that woman and do not imagine as real the life it might have been allowed to lead. For them, the life of the fetus becomes an equally invisible abstraction.[24]

In applying abstract principle to abortion, some insist upon the woman's right since she is a fully developed member of our species, one to whom we grant rights and choices. The fetus, in this argument, is not yet a person equal to all others. It is a part of the woman's biology and outside the sanctity of human life's protection and the law's life interest. If the fetus is one of us, however, its life falls within the protected sphere and must be protected, even at the cost of the mother's right of biological self-determination. These are the only two choices available to us. There is no solution that allows fetus and parent to be seen together not as adversaries but as partners whose social presence is unequal but whose humanity is equally assured. Whatever answer we choose depends on our definitions of humanness and life, on the point we pick along these continuums, and then of subsequent interpretation of both personhood and its resultant rights.

What results is similar to Figure 3.1, an optical illusion. One sees either the white figure or the black, but never the two together. A decision for either parent or fetus necessarily requires the other's rights to be abridged. But abridgment is prohibited because no distinction is allowed between individuals seeking protection or care under the umbrella of their status as sovereign and equal possessors of a citizen's packet of rights. Since choices must be made between competing individuals or classes of individuals whose opposing claims are based upon equal possession of those rights and that membership—the mother and the fetus—one or another party must have its rights restricted. Because we define full membership on the basis of those rights, and the principles that empower them, this denies one or the other standing within our community. Neither these principles nor the logic that applies them, allow mother and fetus to be simultaneously considered.

Euthanasia

The North American debate over the legalization of euthanasia and assisted suicide involves a similar and equally irreducible conflict. Its form

Figure 3.1
Optical Illusion

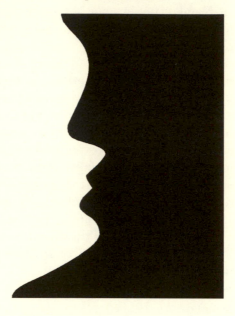

can be stated quite briefly, substituting the fragile patient for the fetus. The principle of biologic self-determination is assumed to include personal choices regarding life and death. Thus every human being has the right to make decisions about his or her termination. But our universal belief in the sanctity of human life principle assures a social protection of human life's continuance. Euthanasia, however, assumes social participation—by medical personnel who will assist in the death, pharmacists who will provide the poison, and society itself that permits the action. We insist upon a principle of nonmalfeasance: "Above all, do no harm," Hippocrates enjoined. And yet, what greater harm is there than to violate human life's sanctity? Finally, many suggest that legalizing euthanasia or assisted suicide will result in unacceptable pressure being placed on the fragile to allow their deaths to be induced,[25] thus violating the injunction of justice and equal protection for all.

In Sorites-like fashion, the question becomes, "when is treatment beneficial, when is it simply murder?" Is it curing or killing to prescribe enough morphine to ease an end-stage cancer patient's pain, even if it may suppress that person's breathing and shorten his or her life by days or weeks? If the answer is that this makes sense, does it also make sense when the pain is not physical but emotional? If we insist upon nonmalfeasance as a principle, are we doing harm by treating a patient's pain or suffering and by that act shortening or ending his or her life, or is harm committed by refusing and thus permitting the physical suffering to continue? No one answer resolves the issue to everyone's satisfaction. No principle adequately serves to untangle the dilemma euthanasia presents.

And so we are caught in logic's two-step shuffle. Where conflicts occur, the first step is to try to redefine the elements of the governing principle in a manner that will resolve the problem. Different principles are applied, each with the same effect. Because each principle is important, none can be set aside. Because all are abstractions, definitions are endlessly debated. What results is an equal claim in a context that demands one or another position, policy, or claimant be chosen. It is at every level the problem of the heap occurs, with stakes far higher than a pile of sand.

METAPROBLEM

What results is a metaproblem based on conflicting principles and their rights applications. The general outline of the problem can be broadly stated in the following manner:

> An individual's or group's inalienable sovereignty—defined as that person's or group's protected range of action—must be restricted to protect another individual or group's equally integral and similarly protected sovereignty. Thus, one or the other must be denied one or more inalienable rights, up to and including the right to life. Since all rights are the reflexive result of species membership, this resolution requires that one or another person or group's full membership be restricted. No such restriction is possible, however, because all members are equal, and all principled rights are to be equally applied. Sovereignty, defined by a shared packet of rights and applicable to all, applies to both the superordinate category of human being and the subordinate category of individual human persons.

We are returned to Tribe's clash of absolutes, to the paradoxical nature of the agreed upon but abstract principle's applicability in one or

Figure 3.2
Facing Illusion

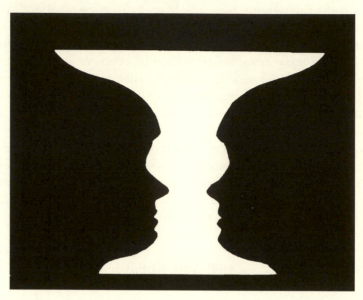

another context requiring that decisions be made. From the perspective of legalists and ethicists, the metaparadox is similar to the famous optical illusion where one can perceive either the outlines of individual faces or the shape of a glass or goblet separating them. But one can never simultaneously see faces and goblet together (see Figure 3.2). The outlined silhouettes represent competing claimants, or classes of claimants, in a rights-based debate or dilemma: fetus versus mother, biological versus adoptive parents, rich versus poor, needy youth versus needy senior, and so forth.

The symmetrical goblet that both separates and defines each pair of claimants represents the set of rights and principles assumed to describe us as a species and thus to apply equally to us all. Administrators of the justice tradition—ethicists, judges, and law makers—are trained to preserve and protect the goblet's shape, assuming the integrity of all claimants will be protected in the process. But it is impossible to bring together the opposing claimants—the silhouettes—without altering the principles that place them in opposition. As a result, we are left with eternal opposition between parties whose perception across the goblet of principled interpretation will admit no resolution.

RESOLUTIONS

It is possible to restate these problems in a way that permits resolution without abandoning all principle, without denying the moral intuitions of persons who must make difficult bioethical choices. Different and apparently conflicting principles can be first focused and then balanced, one with the other. To do so requires a series of transformations that will create a common ground from which the best of traditional bioethics can be preserved within a more concrete, problem-oriented perspective.

First and foremost, the transformational changes require that the principles and values traditionally accepted as a priori ethical truths be reformulated as criteria, as definitions applicable in a specific context. Those criteria must then be applied in a system that permits partial results, one acknowledging the potential for partiality. As Ronald Dworkin points out, principles have a weight and importance that places them in a category of assumed correctness.[26] They are assumed to have a validity that is not to be questioned. But if valued principles have importance it can only be arrived at through questioning and precise definition in a specific context. Unlike principles, criteria are smaller and more malleable constructs susceptible to modification in the face of new data and new problems.

Let us assume that the axiomatic rights historically defined as universal principles at a superordinate level, the level of "human being," do not necessarily serve in any meaningful way as rules operating at the level of the subordinate claimant (fetus, mother, frail elderly patient). Our generalities, in other words, do not address the concrete realities of the dilemmas we face. Thus, in seeking a better methodology for the examination of ethical principles, the scale at which definitions are applied must be a constant consideration.

Second, the operative criteria derived from principle must be seen not as axioms or values that are given, but as goals to be investigated. That is, each criteria must be defined in terms of the value it supposedly represents. If the goal is "justice," for example—an operative principle whose rules govern how we exist together as a group—its reality must be sought not in the broad ideal but in the minutiae of its application. "Justice is found not just in the substantive content" of law and policies, as E. H. Morreim noted, but also in the "procedures by which these are made and managed."[27] After all, "Justice is not only in what the rules say, but in how the rules are made." Thinking first of definitions, second about the methods of their application, and finally of the values they are to represent should assist in defining policies that are consistent, ethical, and comprehensive to all.

In moving from abstract principle to practical criteria, what may be lost is an assumption of universality common to principled argument. What a Canadian in Toronto might see as just and appropriate might be different from what a Hawaiian American would accept. The views of both might diverge radically from the assumptions of a businessman in Canton. Thus, it may not be enough to examine the definition of rules and processes in any one context. It may be that the real challenge ultimately will lie in determining the applicable scale of those definitions and the more general, regional context of their application.

Third, the mechanisms that are used to implement policies and rules must admit to partial membership and to degree. The assumption of absolute categories within bivalent definitions of membership (one is or is not a human being, one is or is not wholly protected) contributes to paradoxical ethics. A better system would permit discussion of degrees of membership within a class and a mechanism of analysis that is multivalent rather than bivalent.

Finally, the restatement of these dilemmas demands a concrete focus in both formulation and application. What, for example, is the issue in the abortion debates? If the issue is protection of human life, as those who oppose the procedure insist, then they seek to foster a quality that extends beyond the pre-born. Where they draw the line between life and nonlife (will they protect those in a permanent vegetative state, for example?) is clearly an issue. However they define it, salvation of the fetus is a subset of a larger goal. Do they fight for those in a persistent vegetative state, for example, or the fragile whose lives may be endangered by the lack of social service and universal medical insurance? Do they oppose the execution of criminals, who are clearly living beings whatever the crimes they may have committed? If one takes them at their word—"We oppose murder!"—the goal of their campaign can't be limited to fetal protection and be consistent.

Similarly, those who insist the issue is a woman's right to self-determination would have trouble finding a concrete and comprehensive statement of their position. At what level is self-determination bounded, for women and for men? None insist, after all, that it is an absolute. For them, as for us all, self-determination does not permit women to choose with impunity to murder, steal, and abandon or abuse the children to whom they give birth. Traditional formulations of this and other problems based on either values (the sanctity of human life) or principles (self-determination) lead to Sorites-style problems. Before they can be re-solved, the problems must be made clear and concrete. The relation between limited cases (the "pre-born") need to be seen as members of greater classes of claimants. The criteria of their definitions need to be clarified and made concrete.

It is possible to construct and then test a set of characteristics that will result in a potentially applicable definition of these problems. It is possible to create a clear definition of what we mean by humanness, or person-hood, and to see what that will mean in terms of inclusiveness and action. The criteria may be discussed independently or with reference to the anencephalic, the PVS patient, the living fetus, or the fragile senior. Such a discussion will make no absolute claims for a specific set of criteria which, as the focus of group discussion, are themselves subject of redefin-ition and analysis.

MULTICRITERION DECISION MAKING

The rest of this book focuses on an approach permitting this type of concrete specificity, a way to rephrase and then test the limits of our assumptions. This approach, called multicriterion decision making (MCDM), is then applied to two critical bioethical problems as a dem-onstration. The data used in this work come from a project completed between 1995 and 1997 as part of a pilot program to test formal multi-criterion decision support approaches in the Department of Bioethics, Hospital for Sick Children, Toronto, Canada. In both cases, the Analytic Hierarchy Process (AHP),[28] one of the best-known multicriterion deci-sion making (MCDM) methods,[29] was utilized in a series of small group sessions composed of hospital employees, involved stake holders (mem-bers of the Down Syndrome Family Association), and a control group of average middle-class citizens interested in, but not professionally involved with, health care issues.

While AHP had not been widely used in the area of bioethics prior to this pilot program, it had been applied extensively in the prioritization and allocation of environmental and other physical resources.[30] It had also been one of the most widely used MCDM methodologies for group decision making[31] and for conflict resolution and consensus-seeking in general.[32] Further, since the AHP is at heart a theory of measurement, it has been used since its inception to develop new scales with which to measure so-called intangibles. Thus, its application to issues involving "human resources" follows a line of theory and practice already well tested in different yet analogous arenas.

The Analytic Hierarchy Process uses a hierarchical structure to formulate and analyze a problem. The overall goal is placed at the top of the hierarchy, with at least one level of criteria beneath it, and with the alternatives (if any) forming the bottom level. Criteria used in a hierarchy may be virtually any relevant decision factor—actors or stakeholders, time periods, causative factors, alternative scenarios—and it is more common than not to have more than one such level. The alternatives are evaluated with respect to the lowest level criteria. Those in turn are assessed with respect to the criteria immediately above them, and so on, until the highest level criteria are evaluated with respect to the overall goal. Finally, all individual evaluations are integrated to yield an overall assessment of their relative importance in the forms of weights, called "priorities," for each alternative. The essence of the approach thus requires the hierarchical decomposition of a complex problem into its relevant aspects, assessment of the options in terms of those aspects, and the aggregation of those individual judgments into an overall measure of the "worth" of each alternative in achieving the goal.

The heart of the AHP is found in its assessment and aggregation procedures, the way it compares criteria and then combines those comparisons. Assessment is made through pairwise comparison of the elements at one level with respect to an element in the level immediately above. Comparison is made in terms of the degree or intensity with which one element dominates the other as regards preference, likelihood, importance, or some similar relevant relation. Dominance may be expressed either linguistically ("Fact A is much more important than Factor B in determining that outcome") or numerically ("Fact A is three times as important as Factor B . . .").

When given linguistically, the expressed intensities are subsequently mapped onto a one to nine numerical scale. From this set of comparisons, various mathematical or statistical procedures can be used to extract weights ("priorities") that represent each element's relative dominance or value. Totaling of the individual priorities ("aggregation") yields an alternative's global priority or dominance, which is effected by multiplying up through the hierarchy and summing the products corresponding to the alternative in question.

While MCDM approaches like the Analytic Hierarchy Process are typically used to determine what political scientists call a "social choice function," it is used here to generate a social preference list, the result of what is sometimes called a "social welfare function."[33] The former accepts as input a sequence of criteria (list A), yielding either a single alternative, "the winner," or a set of winning alternatives. The latter yields a ranking of the set's criterion without identifying a "winner" and thus represents a means of examining the applicability of the criteria and the suitability of individual criteria. The lessons of the last chapter argue against a single criterion, a single principle that will decide or define a problem. What was sought through this approach was a methodology that might balance a range of criteria—clinical, social, and ethical—together.

Obviously, social choice and welfare functions are closely related. Each can be used to create the other. By including "alternatives" at the bottom of a model—for example, levels of care (palliative, stabilizing, ICU, etc.)—the preference list might be transformed into a social choice model defining the best treatment choice. By removing alternatives from a model seeking a single, dominant criterion or treatment approach—a winner—one ends with a social preference list's ranking of preference criteria. The primary goal of these projects was the definition of guidelines and not the selection of individual candidates or treatments. The hierarchies tested were therefore social preference functions. Either approach could have been used, however, to address the central issue, the potential suitability of this type of approach for the evaluation of seemingly paradoxical dilemmas in medical ethics.

While AHP and other similar methodologies are often used either by individual decision makers, or by large single groups of decision makers who are asked to first construct a hierarchy and then to review it, a different approach was utilized in this case. Small focus groups of between five and twelve members met together to evaluate a previously constructed hierarchy describing one or another target issue. Because one aim of the work was to examine existing rules and definitions currently used in medical decision making in specific problem areas, hierarchies were developed for both test problems and then submitted to participants. Both were based on a thorough literature review, each was presented to participating group members for their consideration.

Another goal was to determine the potential for agreement between medical professionals, "normal" citizen, or stakeholders with a vested interest in the problem itself. Thus, to examine the issue of organ transplant eligibility, for example, groups were constituted from three separate communities. The first included hospital-based medical professionals (doctors, nurses, pastoral counselors, bioethicists, social workers, etc.) involved in transplantation issues. The second included members of a Down Syndrome Family Association. Persons with Down syndrome are more prone than those in the general population to conditions requiring transplantation. Finally, a "citizen" group composed of normal members of the community without ties to the hospital or stakeholder groups was created. Members of each group separately considered the same hierarchy. The data returned by the AHP for each group—numerical priorities defining the relationship between criteria in the resulting social choice function— was used to compare and where possible combine the judgments of groups distinguished by professional viewpoint and personal interest.

As the next three chapters make clear, this approach neither restricts ethical decision making to the technically adept nor requires persons to abandon the personal or professional ethical perspectives we all bring to a problem. The hierarchy considered assured, simply, that all discussion was framed by a single set of clearly understood criteria related to a single, clearly definable goal. The system of pairwise comparison assures that in each group discussion of criteria it detailed a quantifiable set of priorities will be returned. Those characteristics facilitated comparison between groups in a way that other more traditional discourse-based approaches to ethics do not. Still, no special claims are made for AHP over other, similar decision-making systems or for multicriterion approaches as a panacea capable of resolving all bioethical dilemmas. The Analytic Hierarchy Process was simply a tool whose methodology focused discussion and whose numerical results facilitated analysis of a specific group's judgments as well as comparison between disparate discussion groups.

In the presentation of this pilot project attention is paid both to qualitative data gathered during group discussions and to the priorities returned by the process of pairwise comparison. Ultimately, the reasons behind judgments articulated in group discussions—the process of moral reasoning in a group context—were as revealing as the final, quantifiable decisions made by group members. As recordings of these sessions make clear, criteria that seemed clear in the literature were critiqued and sometimes rejected by participants who struggled to apply both personal experiences and principles to the pre-selected criteria presented to them. Thus the quantitative results returned by the AHP are interpreted in the context of the deliberations whose result was a series of pairwise comparisons of specific criteria.

4

Absolute Scarcity: Who Gets the Organ Transplant?

In early 1995, Terry Urquart, a person with Down syndrome, was denied a position on the organ transplant waiting list at University Hospital, Edmonton, because he lacked "reasonable" intelligence, a criterion for all prospective organ recipients at that organ transplantation center. Protests by his family and by advocacy groups championing the cause of people with developmental difficulties became a well-photographed story on the nightly television news and one documented by the nation's newspapers.[1] That Terry Urquart was a gold medal skier in the Special Olympics created a story that implicitly questioned the patriotism of the hospital (Urquart represented Canada internationally!), and explicitly, the treatment of all those with developmental difficulties in a critical area of bioethical decision making.[2] Perhaps predictably, given the allegiance of North Americans to successful athletes, the Terry Urquart story became the focus of public debate over the equability and fairness of organ transplantation procedures.[3]

University Hospital was criticized for policies perceived by many as simultaneously arbitrary and prejudicial. This Olympic athlete was as worthy as any transplant candidate, supporters said, whatever his intelligence quotient (IQ). "Shame on those Albertans," a *Toronto Star* reader wrote in a letter-to-the-editor.[4] "Perhaps I should stipulate on my donor card that my organs are to be used for mentally handicapped people only." A child with Down syndrome, is "a living, breathing, human being just like the next child," said another writer. "You wouldn't deny a transplant to a[ny other] child who was otherwise healthy."[5] Because health care is funded by both provincial and federal governments under the Canada Health Act, Terry Urquart's exclusion was seen as a failure of the system at large and not merely a local aberration. "This shameful display of prejudice on the part of our health system must come to an end," said a *Calgary Herald* reader in a letter titled, "Health Service Trying to Play God."[6] Finally, an *Ottawa Citizen* reader asked, in a letter ambiguously titled "Morally Outrageous," "Why would mental capacity of a person be a factor in eligibility for an organ transplant?" In effect he asked: What's so great about intelligence?[7]

Faced with this very public and widespread sentiment—and after several nationally reported rallies in support of Terry Urquart's "right" to "equal treatment"—the hospital reversed its decision, placed the teenager on the transplant waiting list, and removed "reasonable intelligence" as a criterion for eligibility. In its place the hospital substituted a standard of self-sufficiency. It was defined as a person's ability to care for him-or herself, "or failing that, they might qualify with a family [member] capable of doing the job for them."[8] While Terry Urquart's family and supporters were heartened by this decision, public response to this new policy was as negative as it has been to the earlier standard.

These critics argued that candidates with developmental disabilities would not be able to enjoy or "care for" donated organs and would be unable to "repay" the "gift of life" through productive social action. "People said they wanted the organs to go to people who could enjoy their renewed health and who could look after the organs," a hospital spokesperson reported. "It was surprising how overwhelming the reaction was."[9] The general consensus on the part of these critics was that transplant organs should go to those who may live longer and contribute more to society that a person with Down syndrome.[10]

Angered by what they perceived as a "wasting" of valuable organs on a "mentally handicapped" person, some Albertans threatened to tear up their organ donor cards rather than be potential donors to those with developmental challenges.[11] Thus, public backlash threatened to exacerbate the already critical condition of organ scarcity by diminishing the already inadequate pool of potential donors. As one Edmonton physician told reporters, the problem is simple: "There are only enough hearts and lungs to save two of every three people waiting."[12] Where organ donation is voluntary—and especially where public funds are used to support transplantation procedures[13]—broad support of eligibility criteria is a necessity. Any decision made in this context that is unacceptable to the general public has the potential of exacerbating the scarcity of donor organs and thus creating a context for ever more difficult transplant allocation decisions.

Those who looked to medical experts for a definitive answer to this question were disappointed. While IQ is often used as a measure of intelligence in organ transplantation, there is disagreement on both its intrinsic importance and the degree to which it should be employed as a criterion. In a review of international organ transplantation policies, for example, M. E. Olbrisch and J. L. Levenson found a widespread use of IQ as a noncompensatory criteria in some but not all hospitals. And among those surveyed who did use IQ as a criteria in transplant allocation decisions, there was no unanimity regarding the level of intelligence at which it was to be applied or the method by which it was to be measured.[14] Other measures of intelligence and mental competence were even more disputed.

What was meant by intelligence, how it might be measured and its relevance to transplantation was an issue in another very public transplant allocation case. In the summer of 1995, a similar public battle was enjoined in the United States when disabilities activist Sandra Jensen, who required a heart-lung transplant, was denied a place on the organ transplant waiting list because she had Down syndrome. Transplant officials at both UC San Diego and UC Stanford insisted that "Down syndrome patients were not appropriate transplant recipients because they might not be able to mentally negotiate through the complications that could occur after surgery."[15] Like Urquart, Jensen was a public figure, an expert on independent living who had been recognized by, among others, President George Bush in 1990.[16] Unlike Urquart, however, a psychiatric evaluation at UC San Diego determined an "atypically good prognosis" to understand and follow a posttransplant rehabilitation regime.

Finally, in June 1995, public opinion was divided in the United States over the fairness and correctness of providing a liver transplant to Mickey Mantle, a former baseball star and recovering alcoholic, and to actor and former alcoholic Larry Hagman. Mantle received a life-saving liver transplant a day after he was admitted to Baylor University Medical Center in Dallas, Texas. News coverage of Mantle's transplantation emphasized that the average waiting time for a donated liver in many states is at least 140 days, and at least 10 percent of those on the organ transplantation waiting list die before a suitable organ can be found for them.[17] Hagman, on the other hand, who was diagnosed with cirrhosis of the liver in 1992 and had been previously treated for liver cancer, received his new organ after a month-long wait. The average wait, according to transplant registry figures, is at least four months for the average patient.[18]

Because time waiting on an organ transplant list is supposedly a justice criterion assuring that all potential recipients are treated equally on a "first come, first serve" basis, the general perception of Mantle's rapid assignment of a new organ was one of special treatment. Physicians seemed surprised at the controversy surrounding his receipt of an organ in so rapid a manner. Personnel at several United Network for Organ Sharing (UNOS) participating organ transplantation centers explained to journalists that it is not uncommon for patients in dire need to be "jumped to the head of the line." Still, columnists and commentators argued a general perception that Mantle may have received special treatment.[19]

Perhaps more critically, many citizens and medical experts argued that Mantle, a sixty-three-year-old recovering alcoholic, should not have been placed on the waiting list at all. "Spending $300,000 for a liver transplant for someone who's brought harm on himself is not a prudent use of scarce money and scarce livers," Dr. Arthur Caplan, University of Pennsylvania director of the Center for Bioethics, told the Canadian Broadcasting Corporation.[20] Some argued that alcoholics, and by extension others who have contributed to their medically urgent conditions, should be penalized in the organ assignment process. Even if that is true, others said, special consideration for Mantle made sense because, as one University of Chicago ethicist put it, "I think we should give deference to the rare heroes in American Life."[21] "Swell," rejoined *San Francisco Chronicle* columnist Arthur Hoppe. "While thousands of ordinary souls will die for lack of new livers, Mr. Mantle may well have been spared simply because long ago he was good at hitting a ball with a stick. . . . It is those with deep pockets who can purchase more years on this planet."[22]

These cases raise fundamental questions about the uniformity and fairness of the current allocation process. At the same time they appeared to contradict the confident boost of system advocates that, "No part of the health care system has done more to resolve questions of justice than transplantation."[23] Where, some asked, is the justice when aging, alcoholic actors and has-been former athletes receive transplants denied to activists for the disabled and Special Olympics gold medal winners? The range of passions revealed by these debates illustrates the general difficulty of defining allocative criteria in a diverse society. In a country apparently as divided as Canada between those who ask, in effect, "Why waste time on unproductive people?" and those who wonder, "What's so great about intelligence?" the prospect of an enlightened and humane policy acceptable to all parties seems unachievable.

ABSOLUTE VERSUS RELATIVE SCARCITY

Unlike most other areas of bioethical and ethical debate, decisions affecting organ transplantation occur in a context of absolute scarcity, one in which demand far outstrips current or potential supply. This is unusual and perhaps unique. In the more typical condition of relative (sometimes called comparative) scarcity—where resources are at least potentially available—the question is whether society *should* provide care or support to a class of petitioners.[24] In debates on the appropriateness of ventilator support for severely anencephalic infants, for example, the question has never been the availability of stabilizing treatment but whether such procedures should be supported.[25] In the 1970s, the U.S. debate on federal support for renal dialysis turned on the moral obligations of a rich society in a context of relative scarcity, on what *should* be done because it *could* be done.[26]

In the case of organ transplantation eligibility, however, the absolute scarcity of available organs means that some candidates will die no matter what policy is followed. All who are needy cannot be saved. Decisions must be made. As of July 5, 1995, there were 40,989 patients registered on the UNOS organ transplant waiting list, more than double the number of patients who received organ transplants in the whole of 1994.[27] That is to say that, if Terry Urquart or Sandra Jensen got new organs, someone would not. The problem of eligibility could not and cannot be resolved either by increased financial support or official mandate. The dilemma of necessary allocation was and is real.

In the context of absolute scarcity there is no absolute "right" to treatment because a supply of organs necessary for all claimants is unavailable. The Hippocratic Oath's injunction to "do no harm" by definition must be bent because harm necessarily will be done to those potential organ recipients who do not receive a transplant.[28] Principles of the sanctity of life must be violated because some people but not other people will be left to die, and decisions on shortening one or another human life will be made based on considerations of relative merit.[29]

The dilemma of organ allocation thus presents the classic lifeboat problem that has troubled moralists and ethicists ever since an American sailing ship, the *William Brown*, sank in 1841 off the coast of Newfoundland. Crew members rescued many members in a lifeboat captained by the first mate, too many, in fact, to allow the small boat to survive in stormy seas. To assure the survival of some persons, the mate ordered fourteen of those originally rescued out of the lifeboat and into the still stormy sea. While the decision was his, it was one all necessarily agreed to. Ever since that night, the question has been asked: Who is to be sacrificed if others are to live? Is there a humane and responsible way to make such decisions in a context of absolute scarcity?

Like the lifeboat dilemma—is it moral to throw some passengers into the sea so the majority can survive?—the context of absolute scarcity in the realm of organ transplantation challenges our ethical paradigm. As Albertan critics of the policy change at University Hospital made clear, the question of self-interest necessarily dominates when absolute scarcity rules. If a person is too weak to survive the rigors of the lifeboat, or is unable to assist in its maintenance, then their position should go to someone better able both to survive and to contribute to the survival of others in the boat. Traditional guides to moral behavior are, from this perspective, a luxury applicable only when abundance reins.

From this perspective, the debate over the fate of Terry Urquart, and by extension other petitioners in a context of absolute scarcity, is not one that can be resolved by reference to traditional moral language. More simply, it is a question of the scale and nature of our allegiance. We want to save our children, our neighbor's children. But when the person at risk is different from us, an abstraction living far away, then we seek a method to define appropriate behavior in terms of general principles like "good stewardship" or "greatest good." How can the immediate need of the parent and the general needs of society be fairly balanced? What are the individual qualities that create a context of loyalty, which qualify a man or woman to receive a transplant, to stay in the lifeboat, leaving another who will be cast out?

TRANSPLANTATION AND ELIGIBILITY

There are at least two distinct levels at which decisions on organ transplantation allocation are made in North America. First, individual hospitals either accept or refuse candidate placement on the organ transplant waiting list. If they are accepted, there are then a series of criteria administered locally but supervised in the United States nationally through agreed upon protocols. Maintained under federal contract in the United

States by UNOS, these rules rank potential organ recipients on the basis of a supposedly impartial, normative clinical standard designed to balance a number of complimentary, medically relevant factors.[30] This set of criteria is almost universally accepted and has been well described.[31] Similar protocols are used in Canada, which some researchers believe could be efficiently included in the UNOS program, as well as in Western Europe.[32] The 18,251 transplantation procedures performed in 1994 at 278 participating U.S.–based medical institutions operating under the UNOS umbrella can be taken as a measure of the importance of both the program and its criteria.[33]

Normative criteria include urgency of recipient need, defined by a five-point scale; time spent waiting for a transplant, and compatibility between donor organ and prospective recipient (degree of histocompatibility, etc.).[34] Patients who have already rejected a transplant, or who require multiple organ replacement, are deemed less desirable candidates than those waiting for a single organ replacement and have no history of organ rejection.

Table 4.1 presents a previously published summary of this multifactoral, normative approach, with weightings assigned individual criterion through the Analytic Hierarchy Process described below.[35] While it is based on normative criteria for liver transplantation, the model is, with minor changes, applicable to all organ transplant protocols.[36] Graft-preservation time may vary depending on the organ in question, for example, and matching of donor organ to recipient body weight is a criterion critical in some but not all organ transplantation allocation procedures.[37]

All criteria except two define a medically viable match between donor organ and potential recipient. Exceptions are the scale of medical urgency, defining the patient's condition at the time an organ becomes available, and the ranked waiting time on the list of potential recipients. The latter is the system's bow to the justice ideal application of the principle of "first come, first served." It thus supposedly gives precedence to those who have waited longer for transplantation.

The Mantle case made clear that public assumptions of procedural fairness based on rank waiting are inaccurate. Patients determined to be suitable candidates are typically transplanted on a basis of medical urgency—sickest first—with little regard to time spent on the waiting list.[38] Of 162 liver transplant procedures carried out at one transplant center over an eight-month period, "more than two-thirds of the operations were performed after the patients had deteriorated to the point of requiring chronic hospitalization, and in 37.7 percent of the total cases, the recipients had entered the lethal classes five and six from which even short-

Table 4.1
Goal: Transplantation Criteria, Medical

Criteria	Sub-criteria	Sub-criteria (2)
Compatibility (.502)	Adequate (.126) Perfect (.376)	
Medical status (.265)	Urgent (.092)	Urgent stage 3　(.009) Urgent stage 4　(.027) Urgent stage 5　(.037) Urgent stage 6　(.018)
	Replantation (.173)	Primary　(.073) Secondary (.084) Multiple　(.016)
Financial (.065)	No dollars (.005) Dollars (.026) Insurance (.034)	
Waiting (.037)	> 24 Months　(.018) 13-24 months (.026) 7-12 months　(.006) 0-6 months　(.003)	
Logistics (.131)	Graft Preservation (.104)	>20 hours (.008)[+] 11-20 Hours (.020) <10 hours (.076)
	Complexity (.027)	Procedural Difficulty (.005) Routine (.022)

Notes on Individual Criterion

Logistics, *Graft preservation*: Distance between available organ and potential recipient. Organs degrade within hours and must be transplanted within a specific time frame. Logistics: *Complexity*. Difficult as a function of previous, failed transplantation or other complication.
Replantation: single or multiple organ transplant? First or second attempt at transplantation?
Waiting: Time on waiting list.

Based on D. R. Cook et al., A method to allocate livers for orthotopic transplantation: An application of the Analytic Hierarchy Process, *Proceedings of the International Conference on Multiple Criteria Decision Making Applications in Industry and Science*. Asian Institute of Technology, Bangkok, December 6-8, 1989.

Table 4.2
Hierarchy of Allocation Criteria

Histocompatability	.502
Medical status	.265
Logistics	.131
Financial status	.065
Waiting time	.037

term survival was not possible without transplantation."[39] Simply, patients who wait until their medical status is critical are routinely "jumped" to the head of the waiting line, irrespective of social justice promises or concerns.

This is illustrated by relative weightings (Table 4.2) derived from an analysis of allocation criteria assigned by a Pittsburgh University Health Center team of "Surgeons, procurement coordinators, anesthesiologists, transplantation coordinators, financial officers, ethicists, and other interested parties."[40] Once general compatibility between donor organ and recipient is found, medical status is the overwhelming primary consideration in the allocation process. Of all primary criteria in the normative set, time spent waiting was the one least considered by members of that hospital transplant center. In short, despite the public perception of "waiting time" as a just criteria ensuring fairness, it is one devalued if not ignored in actual practice.

If justice and fairness are desirable elements in this process, it would seem that a higher value must be given to "time waiting," irrespective of a competing patient's condition. Were such a change to be made at an organ transplant center, however, it would require physician notification, discussion, and a phasing in period of from one to two years. This would be necessary to assure that patients whose physicians have not entered a patient on the waiting list because they were not yet critical would not be unduly penalized by a late entry and procedural change.

PRESCRIPTIVE CRITERIA

Were transplant centers to make this change, however, it would not address the problem of who should be accepted on the waiting list, an-

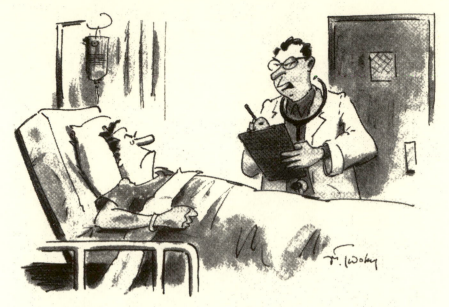

"That liver went to someone who doesn't have such a big yap."

Mike Twohy © 1997 from The New Yorker Collection. All Rights Reserved.

other level of decision making, and what qualities should they possess. After all, the currently accepted, normative set is applied only after a patient is placed on the transplant eligibility waiting list. Whether a patient is accepted or rejected as a candidate for transplantation remains a typically idiosyncratic determination based on the perspective of individual physicians, or at best, the singular policy of an independent organ transplantation center. Should people with largely self-induced conditions—alcoholics with cirrhosis of the liver, for example—be placed on the list? What is "reasonable" intelligence and how should it be evaluated? There is at present neither a set of prescriptive social criteria assuring equal justice in the process of evaluating patients for the transplant eligibility list or a methodology accepted as applicable to this task.

And yet, social worth valuations "have been central in society's allocation of limited medical resources."[41] As others have noted, "Criteria such as the person's relationship to authority figures, past irresponsible behavior, and intelligence . . . [t]he patient's marital status, number of dependents, income, educational background and employment record were all evaluated to determine the patient's potential to return to a 'productive life' [after a transplant]."[42] Loosely grouped under the heading of "psychosocial" eligibility,[43] prescriptive criteria may include prior health or social habits (alcoholism, for example), chronological age, social standing, and other nonmedical standards. In some cases, emotional stability has been suggested as a determining prescriptive criteria.[44] In the United States, both citizenship (or legal residency)[45] and a potential organ recipient's ability to pay for services—alone or through an insurer—are also considerations determining patient eligibility.

It is at this stage of the process that the veneer of equitable treatment and justice necessary to the process at large most obviously breaks down. At the worst, the specter of two classes of citizen, those who are "donors" and those who would be recipients, is created. Donor classes would include, for example, anencephalic infants[46] and patients with developmental disorders—Down syndrome, for example—whose organs are sought as a resource but who are themselves barred from receiving organs by reason of their infirmities.[47] Various areas have reported a consistently larger number of organ donors of color relative to the dominant Caucasian population. This follows a general rule of resource allocation, noted by some critics, that the most disadvantaged receive the least care at every level.[48] Recipient classes would include those who are wealthy, white, and otherwise socially acceptable, whatever the cause of their condition or relative potential for survival. With the perspective of such a division, the concept of equitable, distributive justice becomes an empty hope.

MULTICRITERION APPROACHES

The question then becomes how to describe a set of prescriptive criteria that will be accepted as fair and equitable by both medical professionals and the general public whose voluntary participation in organ donation programs provides the critical basis of transplant organ supply. A list of criteria defining eligibility for the transplant organ waiting list must be compatible with both normative criteria (Table 4.1) and social values active in a context of absolute scarcity. Ideally, the set should be at least as precise and nonjudgmental as the one now defining normative judgments. Because transplant organ supply depends on the willing and unremunerated participation of potential donors, the set must have public input to assure public support. Without it, there is the risk—as the Urquart case demonstrated—of disgruntled potential donors withdrawing their participation.

Any system attempting to define the rules of transplant eligibility must be able to handle a plethora of values and criterion rules defining the final allocative judgment. In the Mickey Mantle case, for example, issues raised were potential for posttransplant survival (Mantle's history of cancer), public recognition of the potential transplant patient (his status as a "hero"), and the origin of his liver problem (alcoholism). For Sandra Jensen, public service and public recognition were balanced against her cognitive limits and their potential relation to her value as a person as well as her ability to follow rigorous posttransplant medical and pharmacological regimes.

A multicriterion approach is particularly appropriate to this type of problem because of its underlying assumptions concerning the way we perceive and resolve complex issues. First, it assumes that few decisions are made on the basis of a single quantifiable criterion. More typically, two or more sometimes competing criteria are required to describe a problem and thus must be compared before a decision can be made. The Analytic Hierarchy Process is an MCDM system designed to generate and analyze an interrelated set of distinct and seemingly unrelated criteria, of "apples and oranges," in the words of one focus group participant.

Second, MCDM approaches generally recognize that "if anything is valued at all, it is valued for more than one reason."[49] Criteria are valued not for themselves, in other words, but as surrogates for the capacities and abilities they supposedly represent. If those are not reflected by a specific criterion—or are deemed irrelevant to the greater problem—then reliance on that criterion will not be merely ineffective, but also counterproductive. Consider the use of IQ as a criterion in organ transplant decision making. It measures a specific type of analytic intelligence. But it may or may not adequately measure a person's ability to understand the gravity of the transplant procedure. It may or may not define a person's ability to follow rigorous posttransplant dietary and pharmacological regimes. It may or may not reflect a social bias against those who while able in many ways will still score poorly on this test. Indeed, as Martin S. Pernick points out, its development earlier in this century was encouraged by eugenics advocates as a tool to combat the "menace of the feeble minded."[50]

Because the focus group methodology using AHP requires participants to compare and then rate the importance of individual criteria against each other, it effectively demands of participants that they consider the applicability and meaning of each criterion. Practically, this means that focus group members discussing criteria must pay equal attention to their representative value ("What does IQ measure, and why is it important here?") and their relative importance (Is this more important, less important, or equal to, say, "survival"?) in choosing between two criteria. Thus, it was hoped that at the least this process would provide a critique of criteria chosen as well as a ranking of their relative importance.

ELIGIBILITY CRITERIA

It was for this reason that the AHP-based hierarchy was constructed from a review of the technical literature and an analysis of news stories covering Canadian and U.S. transplantation controversies. If presented by participants with a hierarchy based upon available literatures, it was hoped that a critical discussion of generally accepted criteria would result. Another approach would have been to ask focus groups to first generate a hierarchy and then to evaluate it. This would have resulted in a series of independent criterion lists and judgments, to be compared, analyzed, and regularized.

Whether or not it would have resulted in better discussion is also unclear. By presenting a completed hierarchy, no participant was particularly vested in any single criterion as "his" or "hers." Thus, nobody felt obliged to defend one or another position because, "Hey, that's mine! I recommended it." This assured that in pairwise comparisons persons were free to question both the meaning and relative importance of all criteria included in the hierarchy. In addition, by providing a literature-based hierarchy, any potential animosity on the part of stakeholder and citizen groups toward hospital personnel was deflected. Criterion were independent of local actors, and the possibility that one or another person might argue against a criterion because it was championed by a disliked colleague—or because the hierarchy itself was generated by one or another hospital group—was avoided.

A tentative hierarchy thus was developed based on a review of the medical literature involving transplantation and eligibility criteria. News stories, editorials, and letters to the editor involving transplant eligibility decisions in the cases of Mickey Mantle, Larry Hagman, Sandra Jensen, and Terry Urquart were also studied. These were used both as a way of reviewing the completeness of the literature-based hierarchy and as general case studies to be discussed as examples, if necessary, in individual discussion groups. This preliminary set was then submitted to bioethicists at The Hospital for Sick Children (Toronto, Canada), for review. Following minor modifications of the hierarchy to reflect local conditions in a pediatric facility, an amended set of six level-1 criteria—each with its own set of defining subcriteria—was organized into an AHP-style hierarchy. Criteria used in this program are presented in Table 4.2. Definitions of the individual criteria employed include:

Intelligence Measured by IQ

While supporters of Sandra Jensen and Terry Urquart insisted intelligence levels should not be a barrier to their eligibility, IQ is a commonly used criterion in organ transplant eligibility standards at the Hospital for Sick Children and elsewhere. A survey of physicians involved in heart transplantation found a pattern of increasing use of an intelligence criteria as IQ declined.[51] Thus while only 25.6 percent of U.S. programs considered an IQ between seventy and fifty points an absolute contraindication to transplantation, 74.4 percent believed an intelligence measured as lower than fifty points an absolute bar to transplantation. Its general and local use clearly required that intelligence measured by IQ be included in this hierarchy.

Long-Term Survival

Transplant organs should go to those who may live longer than the presumably fragile Down syndrome person, some Albertans said. Certainly, given the absolute scarcity of available kidneys, lungs, and hearts, to transplant an organ to a person with a chronic and rapidly terminal condition would seem wasteful. But as others have pointed out, the power of future probabilities diminishes the farther forward they are projected.[52] A limit of ten years following transplantation was chosen for this exercise as the farthest forward that can be projected. The question then becomes first, the degree to which long-term survival is a factor in waiting list eligibility, and second, when it becomes a critical element in decision making.

Social Independence Posttransplant

Some argue that physically self-reliant persons who do not need social support should receive priority in this process. Reflecting that assumption, Alberta hospital officials substituted a criteria of "independence" or "self-sufficiency" for those defining reasonable intelligence. In their construction, independence can refer to either the candidate's ability to physically maintain his or her own existence, or the presence of another person qualified, able, and willing to assist in the maintenance of the patient. The question then, is whether a patient will be able to maintain him or herself, (1) without any support, (2) with the assistance of others, (3) through support of an insurer, or (4) only at public expense.

Physical Activity Posttransplant

Those opposed to Terry Urquart's candidacy insisted he would not be able to "use" the organ sufficiently, that his level of activity was necessarily diminished because of his condition. The normative scale of medical urgency criteria provides a general gross measure of activity, which can be projected forward as the expected patient state following a transplant. These include six distinct ability levels: (1) working (at office or in school); (2) homebound but independent; (3) homebound and requiring support; (4) hospital or institutionally bound, but not in intensive care (ICU); (5) ICU care; and (6) ICU care requiring continuous ventilation or other life sustaining treatment.

Productivity

Will the patient be able to participate in and contribute to society? In recent transplant cases this has normally been defined in terms of public recognition. Terry Urquart was a gold medal skier, internationally recognized for that achievement. Sandra Jensen was a nationally recognized advocate for the disabled person's right to independent living. Larry Hagman was an internationally recognized actor. Thus a scale based on recognition of achievement was used to measure this criterion.

Social Function

We can conceive of a descending scale of social contribution, with the highest level representing individuals whose contributions are recognized internationally. Mother Theresa was frequently mentioned in focus groups as exemplifying extreme selflessness, for example. Those who are active at the community or regional levels would constitute a second level of social function, and so forth. The final step on the five-level scale would be an antisocial person without clear social participation or ties.

Compliance

Patient compliance or noncompliance with medical regimes is a frequently cited criterion in organ transplant allocation discussion.[53] The assumption is that noncompliant patients—those who do not follow medical directives—will not follow rigorous posttransplant medication regimes and will therefore have a higher level of organ rejection. It is often coupled with intelligence levels when a person is believed to lack the mental capacity to understand and follow medical directions. Sandra Jensen's candidacy, for example, was rejected at first by the University of California medical schools on the assumption that as a person with Down syndrome she "might not be able to mentally negotiate through the complications that could occur after surgery."[54]

Patient Responsibility

Public concern, on the other hand, has focused on patient responsibility as a contributing factor to a medical condition requiring organ transplantation. Some suggested, for example, that alcoholics and smokers should be penalized in the allocation procedure because their conditions result, at least in part, from conscious self-abuse.

Because the client population at the target hospital was pediatric, however, the issue of responsibility was seen as largely irrelevant to the staff's deliberations. While adolescents may have some responsibility for their conditions, hospital bioethicists argued that patient responsibility for chronic illness is rarely an issue in this branch of medicine. Thus, while excluded as a criterion in these deliberations, it would be included in a hierarchy discussed at an adult transplant center.

TESTING

Three target groups were then identified in discussion with Hospital for Sick Children bioethicists. They were: (1) hospital staff members involved with its transplant program, (2) nonprofessional community stakeholders with a personal interest in organ transplantation issues, and (3) at least one "control group" of community members uninvolved in either hospital activities or transplantation advocacy. Health professionals were chosen because it is they who care for patients and who today make decisions on eligibility. Stakeholders were included because of their personal interest and involvement. After all, when lawsuits are launched or public protests begun, it is this type of group more than others who will likely be involved. Finally, a group of average, hopefully representative citizens was included as a control group because suitable organs are considered a "public resource," not a commodity. Thus, this group was seen as representative of the society that ultimately has responsibility for distribution of graft organs.

Within the hospital, potential candidates for a transplant eligibility focus group included: physicians (neonatologists, psychiatrists, pediatricians, surgeons, family physicians), nurses, bioethicists, pastoral counselors, and transplant administrators. A hospital bioethicist identified and then invited representatives of each group to participate in this project. Eventually, two hospital-based focus groups were constituted.

Through the Toronto-based Advocacy Resource Centre for the Handicapped (ARCH), members of the Niagara Falls Down Syndrome Family Association were asked to participate in a focus group on transplant eligibility. Members of this group had earlier approached ARCH lawyers to express their concerns over the possible exclusion of persons with Down syndrome from regional transplant programs. That concern was generated both by publicity given to the Terry Urquart case and a local case then being considered by the Ontario Human Rights Commission. In addition, members of the association viewed issues involving organ transplantation within the broader history of discrimination against persons with Down syndrome.

Until quite recently, persons with Down syndrome were devalued by many medical practitioners. Often, they were not treated aggressively as infants for congenital heart defects, a fact that has led to a greater than average need for heart and heart-lung transplants by members of the Down syndrome population. Members of the association thus saw issues of transplant eligibility as critical both practically and in terms of the general goal of equal treatment for persons with this condition. In December 1996, a five-hour session was held with eleven members of the Niagara Falls association, participants being chosen by the association itself. They included parents of Down syndrome persons (homemakers, office workers, several self-employed persons, two nurses) and a man in his thirties with Down syndrome.

Finally, a discussion group involving representatives, middle-class citizens from the Toronto Beaches community was constituted. It was to serve as a "control" group of average citizens whose judgments might be used as a measure for both professional and stakeholder perspectives. Participants included high school teachers, homemakers, a commercial video producer, a landscape gardener, and a freelance writer. The Toronto Beaches community was chosen as a matter of convenience. It is where I live and thus where I could impose on neighbors and acquaintances for help in this project. Thus all participants were known to me—if not to each other—and had expressed a general interest in the issues of health care and were willing to make themselves available for an evening discussion group.

Before each session, participants of all groups were given a handout summarizing the general issues of organ transplant eligibility. With this handout were a list of criteria, which were defined individually and then summarized in a hierarchical table (Table 4.3). Also in the briefing packet was a short description of AHP, including examples of pairwise comparisons using Table 4.2 criteria. Stressed in the preparatory materials was the need for free and frank discussion of issues and the fact that "no one person has all the answers. No one criterion will necessarily dominate. The intent is to discover, through this process, how persons perceive the range of issues considered by many to be important in making these determinations."

It took between three and four hours for the hospital and citizen groups to complete the Analytic Hierarchy Process' pairwise comparisons of the hierarchy's criteria. Down Syndrome Family Association participants required more than five hours to complete the process. The additional time was largely due to an intense, forty-five minute discussion of the relative importance of extremely high IQ when compared with other IQ scores. Hospital groups were broken into two two-hour sessions because of the time constraints of staff members. All other groups met for a single session broken by one or two rest breaks.

For the sake of consistency, I served as the sole moderator for all groups. This meant announcing the pairwise questions, previously loaded into the Expert Choice program, and then asking each participant for his or her initial opinion on each question. Discussion then was open until a "vote" was called. Then each participant again was asked for his or her opinion. While all sessions were tape recorded with the permission of participants, each individual judgment also was manually written down. This served as insurance against a possible tape recorder malfunction and as a way of "ending" each discussion. After each set of comparisons, individual judgments were manually noted, averaged, and then entered into the Expert Choice program. Once a decision was reached and entered into the computer, the discussion could continue.

Table 4.3
Prescriptive Criteria for Organ Transplantation Candidacy

GOAL	CANDIDACY requirements for Transplant Waiting List
CRITERIA	sub-criteria
Intelligence (measured by IQ)	genius (>140 IQ) gifted (115-140 IQ) normal (80-115 IQ) diminished (55-80 IQ) low (< 55 IQ)
Likelihood of Post-transplant survival	10 Years + 5-10 years 3-5 years 1-3 years < 1 year
Social Independence (post-transplant)	will be wholly self-sufficient will need family support will need insurer support will need social assistance will require combination 2-5
Physical Activity Level (post-transplant)	Working (office, school) Home bound but independent Home bound, requiring care Hospital bound, stable ICU bound ICU bound with life support systems
Productivity/Participation	Superior: International recognition Excellent: National recognition Average: productivity/participation Below Average: Minimal/Neutral Negative productivity
Social Function	Superior: the "saint" extreme selflessness Excellent: Community participation Average: "average" community activity Below Average: Asocial person Negative: anti-social person
Patient participation	Compliance (with medical directives) - full compliance with staff directives - partial compliance with staff directives - wholly non-compliant Responsibility (for condition): *excluded from pediatric model.*

Frankly, this was a charade. Persons needed to "see" that a question was completed and that a decision had been made before comfortably moving onto the next question. After the session was completed, however, all individual judgments were entered into an Excel software spreadsheet, the geometric mean of the group's answers to each question was calculated, and this number was then entered into the Expert Choice program. The geometric mean was used as a more reliable means of aggregating group decisions. The Expert Choice software then calculated a final set of relative values for each criteria in the hierarchy. It was these results that were used for cross-group comparison and aggregation.

In analyzing the results, the transcripts of the discussions—or the handwritten notes taken during discussion—were extremely useful. Where differences between groups were evident—for example, in defining the importance of "compliance"—it was only through a review of the group's deliberations that those differences could be understood. In some cases numerical differences between judgments within a group—or between focus groups—did not necessarily reflect vastly different perspectives. Rather, a study of the group transcripts revealed they were the result of different definitions that could be justified in the final analysis.

5

What's So Great about Intelligence?: Focus Group Deliberations

Consensus is the holy grail of liberal ethics, "the touchstone of truth and the guarantor of correctness in matters of belief and of adequacy in matters of decision and action."[1] Its efficacy and its potential are principles cherished by ethicists and bioethicists, who are convinced that through group discourse, truth or its approximation can be discovered in unanimity. Dilemmas would disappear and paradoxical formulations evaporate if only everyone agreed upon the nature of the problems we face and upon the mechanisms that would best resolve them. Indeed, some perceive consensus as a necessary mechanism for resolving uncertainty across the plain of a liberal democracy[2] As Mark Kuczewski says in his review of Jonathan D. Moreno's 1995 book on bioethics and consensus *Deciding Together*, "Liberal democracy requires consensus because moral uncertainty must be managed."[3] From this perspective, the imperative to consensus in bioethics is a subset of the greater mechanisms by which democratic society defines an appropriate position in areas of persistent disagreement.

In bioethics, as in democracy at large, some argue that only consensus built upon discussion can lead to the resolution of the moral and social concerns that are its focus. Consensus-based decision making is, its advocates insist, the last, best hope for those who seek an informed and acceptable resolution to the dilemmas that face us. The assumption that general agreement represents shared standards is the hidden assumption of much modern social science. Focus groups represent one attempt to achieve consensus through discussion. Further, the widespread use of pop-

Figure 5.1
All Groups: Level-1 Criteria

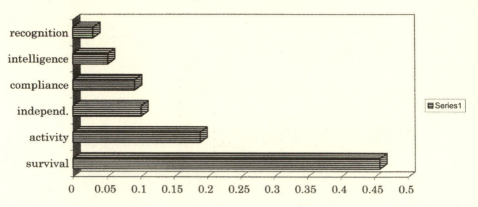

ular polls is assumed, at heart, to measure consensus or its failure. Professional surveys like those cited in the previous chapter at heart are a way to seek professional consensus as a yardstick of correct professional behavior, and of truth. "I'll play your game," one doctor said at the beginning of a focus group on organ transplant allocation issues, "but if you want to know the answers, I've got the papers here." He pointed to a stack of journal articles with data from international surveys of physicians involved in transplantation. In the end, however, it wasn't that simple.

And yet the failure of consensus in some contexts, and the sometimes disastrous results where it has been achieved—for example, Germany in the 1930s—has lead others to doubt its potential. "Consensus," as Nicholas Rescher insists, for example, "can be and often is no more than an agreement in folly."[4] The best that can be hoped for, he argues, is a mechanism that limits conflict when unresolvable disagreements inevitably occur. Participants in the focus groups discussing organ transplant allocation criteria demonstrated that consensus—or at least strong unanimity—is neither impossible nor in its conclusions necessarily foolhardy. Their apparent agreement masks, however, a rich complexity that says much about both the problem at hand and the assumptions inherent in the approach itself.

OVERVIEW

Figure 5.1 offers a graphic illustration of the cumulative, relative ranking of level-1 criteria for all groups. This says very little about consensus,

Figure 5.2
Inconsistency Index

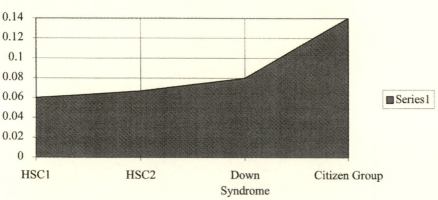

however. It simply summarizes the decisions of all group participants without reference to areas of disagreement or disparity. Still, it is useful. The probability of posttransplant survival is clearly the single most critical criterion to all groups. Level of expected posttransplant activity, a quality of life criterion, is second, and with level of posttransplant social independence apparently qualifying survival as an independent value. Degree of patient compliance and patient intelligence measured by IQ tests clearly are devalued here, especially when compared with the level of widespread usage noted in the last chapter in international surveys. Finally, public recognition—an issue raised by the transplantation of Mickey Mantle—is given only minimal weight in these results.

We can measure the internal consistency of these decisions, group to group and for the focus group program as a whole. What this reports on is the unity of judgments, the apparent integrity of the vision of discussants. Using a consistency index built into the Expert Choice software, each group's cumulative response was measured against randomly generated numbers as a way of judging their internal coherence. If answers are extremely inconsistent, greater than .10, then the assumption is either that there is a problem with the hierarchy or the group considering it may for some reason lack the basis for making appropriate judgments regarding a specific goal. Scores below .10 are generally considered to be within acceptable parameters. Relative scores of all participant groups are given in Figure 5.2.

Both hospital groups were extremely consistent in their judgments, returning scores of .06 and .067, respectively. The Down Syndrome As-

Figure 5.3
Group Summary

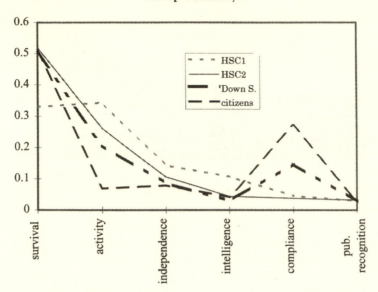

sociation group's index of consistency was slightly higher, measuring .08 on the consistency index. The citizen control group, on the other hand, demonstrated an apparently unacceptable level of inconsistency in their judgments. Within these groups, consistency of judgment clearly decreases as one moves from hospital-based medical professionals to stakeholders with an interest in transplantation and from them to the general lay person.

Detailed analysis presented later in this chapter suggests that the problem presented by the citizen's group's inconsistency does not represent simply a lack of information or citizen group ignorance. The importance assigned by that group to one criteria, "compliance," was almost solely responsible for its unacceptably high ranking in this area. The importance assigned that same criterion by the Down syndrome group also affected its overall consistency. Put another way, had these groups devalued compliance as a criterion, the range of their judgments would have been far more consistent.

Figure 5.3 presents a clearer portrait of areas of agreement and disagreement for level-1 criteria, broken down by groups. Strong consensus reigns in the evaluation of four criteria—survival, social independence, intelligence measured by IQ, and public recognition. The importance of "physical activity" is modestly contested and opinion on "compliance" as a criterion clearly divided. The value of the lay persons group within this program, and of their judgments, will become evident when those criterion are discussed. First, however, it is worthwhile to see where unanimity was reached.

Survival

Survival—the probability a candidate would live through a transplant operation and the period of postoperative adjustment—was the most important criterion determining whether or not a person should be placed on the posttransplant eligibility list. Across the groups, judgments comparing survival to all other criteria were consistently among the strongest choices recorded. "As long as you survive, you have a chance," said one person in the Down Syndrome Family Association group. "If you're dead, you don't." "It doesn't make sense to me to give an organ to someone who is only going to live for a short time," said a member of the citizen review group.

Among members of the hospital groups, survival of both the patient and the transplanted organ was perceived as the essence of both good medicine and good stewardship. Defining viable transplant available organs as a rare, precious resource, members of these groups said their primary responsibility is to assure the organ's continuance in a patient whose life is most likely to be prolonged as a result of a successful transplant procedure.

Members of one hospital group (HSC1) ranked survival slightly behind physical activity, however, insisting that survival meant not bare existence but continuance with a greater than minimal level of postoperative physical function for the host. If raw survival is wholly separated from levels of physical activity a transplant might go to a person who is in a coma, commented one person. That, discussants agreed, would not be good stewardship. Members of other groups were able to separate these two criteria, while agreeing with HSC1's general position that "survival must mean survival with some quality of life." In discussing physical activity, members of HSC1, the Down syndrome and citizen groups all strongly devalued cases of extreme physical limitation, arguing it should be an absolute contraindication in and of itself. A patient in intensive care requiring life support, for example, was seen as so frail as to be an unacceptable candidate.

Figure 5.4
Survival by Years

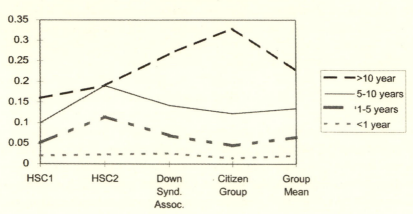

In defining what they meant by survival in terms of years, data summarized in Figure 5.4, participants in all groups agreed that a patient with a probability of less than one-year posttransplant survival was an unlikely candidate for a scarce donor organ. "One year is such a short time and you're spending most of it adjusting to the surgery, and your family is going through these adjustments," said a participating bioethicist. "The burdens seem to outweigh the benefits." Others agreed that the months immediately following a transplant—a period marked by issues of medication, diet, and life-style as well as surgical recovery—is extremely difficult.

That said, members of both hospital groups ranked survival of five to ten years and more than ten years as nearly equal. This reflected, they said, the difficulty of long-term prognosis, their experience in the complications and challenges facing a posttransplant person. It also signals the experience of some who believed even midterm survival may be a worthwhile goal in some cases. A staff psychiatrist, for example, mentioned a case known to her colleagues of a person whose posttransplant complications resolved into "one wonderful year" for a patient who later died. Simply, in the arena of those who spend their working lives with extremely ill patients, seven, five, or even three years may represent a sufficiently rich and meaningful period of time to justify transplantation.

Members of both the Down Syndrome Family Association and the citizen groups generally valued long-term (more than ten years) over mid- and short-term survival rates. It was, they said, the "best bang for the buck" from a scarce resource. They assumed in their discussions that long-term survival was predictable, that in deciding who would be placed on the organ transplant waiting list that long-term survival was a firm criterion. Like hospital personnel, they also devalued shorter survival times, arguing strongly that a survival rate of a year or less would be an absolute contraindication barring eligibility.

While the dominance of survival as a criteria in organ transplant eligibility seems self-evident, it in fact represents a major shift in policy. Historically, in both Canada and the United States, "treatment decisions were made by considering only what was best for each individual."[5] A patient needing an organ might be considered transplant eligible irrespective of his or her potential for long-term survival. For example, Mickey Mantle's liver transplantation was ordered despite a medical history of alcoholism and cancer, which together suggested a poor probability of long-term posttransplant survival. Similarly, strongly ranking survival as a primary criteria would have improved the candidacies of Down syndrome Sandra Jensen and Terry Urquart, both of whom had positive long-term prognoses when they were first denied placement on the eligibility list.

In late 1996 the United Network for Organ Sharing (UNOS) announced policy changes emphasizing survival as a critical, principal criterion in liver transplantation.[6] UNOS controls the allocation of organs for transplantation in the United States and is under contract to the U.S. Department of Health and Human Services. In emphasizing long-term survival, UNOS officials stated they were attempting to recognize the best use of scarce resources and thus to define a principle of good stewardship. As Barbara Ott noted in a review of a preliminary report on these focus groups, both this policy change and the reasoning behind it was anticipated by our focus groups, and thus may serve as an independent verification of their judgment.[7]

Public Recognition

There was also consensus across all groups devaluing public recognition of individual achievement as a criterion for organ transplantation. In all groups the criterion public recognition was consistently and strongly denied as a criterion for admission to the organ transplant waiting list. While members of all groups agreed that, ideally, persons extremely valuable to society in theory should be given priority over those who do not contribute to society, none believed fame or notoriety were reliable indicators of public worth. Further, none knew how to measure this variable or to define the truly critical persons in a society at any time.

For these Toronto groups, favoring the well known also was seen as antithetical to the national health care system's ideals. "Our whole [Canadian health care] system was developed to treat people equally in hospitals," said one member of the citizen group. "Not that it has ever happened, but it's what we try for." This was a consistent theme across the groups. The Canadian health system is in principle dedicated to the ideal of equal service to all persons irrespective of social position or economic need. To value one person over another on the basis of social worth—whether measured by public recognition or some other index— is thus a violation of a deeply held, social tenant in Canada and was rejected as such by all group members. While many believed current changes in health care funding and organization endanger the principle, its value remained operative and critical to members of these groups.

Participants in each group independently framed their discussion of this criterion in terms of one or another well-known public case. Most used the then recent debate over Mickey Mantle's liver transplant as a concrete example of transplantation based on public recognition. Whether the subject was retired baseball players (Mantle), amateur athletes (Terry Urquart), aging actors (Larry Hagman), or social activists (Sandra Jensen), there was an overwhelming skepticism of the use of fame as a social worth indicator. "With Mickey Mantle's [social] contribution," said one woman in the Down Syndrome Association discussion group, "it may be perceived by [my husband] John, a sport's fan, as monumental. But to me, I couldn't care less. And the same with my [Down syndrome] son. His contributions to me, to what I see him doing at school or in the community, I think are quite monumental. But people who don't know him . . ."

Others noted that this type of social worth criterion usually describes past work, not present social activity or the potential of future contributions. "To be crude," said one citizens group participant about Mantle, "his contribution to society had come to an end. I don't want to give him credit [as a transplant candidate] for his past accomplishments." If public recognition or social participation are to be critical issues, in other words, past achievement should not be considered because it is not necessarily a guide to a candidate's potential for future contribution. Thus, just as survival is a forward looking criterion defining stewardship in terms of the survival of both patient and organ, so too must any "social worth" consideration be a matter not simply of past performance but also, and more importantly, a measure of future contribution.

The consensual devaluation of public recognition strongly rejects the arguments of those who supported Mickey Mantle's candidacy. Dr. Mark Siegler, for example, argued that Mantle's transplantation was deserved despite his history of alcoholic cirrhosis and cancer because the baseball legend "is a real American hero who captures the imagination of a generation through his skill and ability and personality." A director of the University of Chicago's clinical ethics program, he told *New York Times* reporter Gina Kolata that, "I think we have to give deference to the rare heroes in American life . . . we have got to take them with all their warts and failures and treat them differently."[8] While recognizing the importance of role models to society—"We need our heroes," said one citizen participant—all agreed that status should not be a lever for special advantages in medical care.

In the same vein, all agreed that while Sandra Jensen and Terry Urquart should not have been denied a place on the organ transplant lists because of their Down syndrome, neither should they have been advanced because of their public position. This, too, was at variance with the official public view. News stories detailing Sandra Jensen's fight for placement on the transplant eligibility list emphasized her past activism and social importance. "Sandra Jensen is nationally recognized for her work helping others with Down syndrome live useful, productive lives," began one story on her fight for placement on a transplant eligibility waiting list.[9] News stories and editorial letters concerning Terry Urquart's candidacy in Canada focused on his winning of a gold medal in the Special Olympics downhill ski competition.[10] To members of the Toronto discussion groups, however—including the Down Syndrome Family Association participants—these issues were deemed as irrelevant as Mickey Mantle's past prowess in deciding a patient's eligibility for organ transplantation.

Since the death of Mickey Mantle, the decision to provide the former baseball player with a liver despite his extremely poor, long-term prognosis has been almost universally condemned. Despite Dr. Siegler's defense of heroes as special cases in medical decision making, transplant professionals have generally rejected the provision of a liver for a recovering alcoholic with cirrhosis of the liver and a recent history of cancer. Similarly, while many applauded the eventual placement of both Jensen and Urquart on organ candidacy lists, no article did so on the basis of their past public service. Rather, their eventual acceptance was seen instead as removing a prejudicial barrier against the cognitively challenged rather than advancing the cause of the publicly recognized. Thus, the views of the group participants seems to be confirmed by a general and official perspective arising from these contentious public cases: Public recognition should no more serve as a criterion for the allocation of scarce transplant organs than social prejudice should be allowed to prevent it.

One exception was made by discussion group members, however. While all refused to distinguish between candidates on the basis of positive public recognition, they did argue that persons convicted of violent crimes should be disqualified as transplant candidates. "If you mean is it between a Mother Theresa and a Paul Bernardo [A famous serial killer in Ontario]," said one hospital staff person, "then, yeah. I'd give it to her." The taking of another's life or the commission of a violent act against another was, in short, a counterindication in the context of absolute scarcity defining organ transplant allocation.

Intelligence

Also strongly devalued as a criterion by members of all groups was intelligence measured by IQ. This is surprising and notable given the widespread use of intelligence measured by IQ as a primary criterion in transplant eligibility decision making. Acknowledging its use at the Hospital for Sick Children, members of both hospital groups said they understood its attraction: "At least with intelligence [measured by IQ] you know that it's not going to change," said one physician. In short, in an area of moral and ethical judgment rife with uncertainty, IQ is a firm number that can be grabbed, pointed to, and used to make an "impartial" judgment that is easily defended.

That said, however, members of all groups insisted that it is neither a guarantor of compliance in posttransplant behavior—one argument sometimes cited for its use—nor an adequate measure of individual abilities. "I guess it's not clear that you need it as an independent criterion," suggested one medical resident assigned to the transplant team, "if you have got a capacity to be compliant, capacity for independent living, an emotional stability to tolerate the procedure . . . if you've got all those, I'm not sure you need it [IQ] independently."

Others went further, insisting that IQ scores do not measure what is important in a person and therefore in a transplant candidate. "In terms of value judgments," said one doctor, "I would think that involvement with others, ability to participate in society and to have a meaningful life would be more important than how you score on an IQ test." Nor was it perceived by these persons as a necessary measure of an individual's ability to follow medical directives or understand necessary posttransplant medication regimes. Thus, among hospital-based participants IQ was seen as an unreliable and insufficient substitute for other criteria defining individual worth through social relation.

Participants in the citizen and Down syndrome association groups agreed. "For me, IQ is not a very important thing by any means," said one woman in the control group. A man whose views were closely listened to by the group at large remarked that, "IQ doesn't measure what this individual gives to other individuals around him or her. It's an arbitrary measure, at best." Indeed, most were surprised to see IQ listed as a criterion in the hierarchy. "They use IQ even though it's been discredited over recent years, it's cultural biases and everything?" asked one woman in the citizens group, shaking her head.

Although IQ was generally devalued as a criterion, participants were still faced with deciding the point where, to the extent it was used at all in decision making, IQ would be considered. While most labeled midrange IQ levels—those between "genius" and "diminished" levels—of nearly equal relevance (or irrelevance), in all groups the majority of participants argued that those with extremely high IQ scores (above 140 basis points) and very low scores (below 50 points) should be considered separately. "This is the hardest question we have to face tonight," said a member of the Down Syndrome Family Association. He argued with his colleagues for forty-five minutes before they agreed with him that the "rare genius," a person with an IQ over 145 points, should be given special consideration. "We've spent our whole lives fighting to be equal," complained the mother of a Down syndrome person, "and then there is this issue." In the end, they concluded that in the very rare cases where a very high IQ score offered the potential social service of extremely rare intellectual ability, that society's needs for its very, very brightest outweighed the egalitarian perspective and the social values this and other groups otherwise espoused. "After all," remarked one participant to the amusement of all, "in Canada we need all the genius we can get."

A similar position was taken by one of the two hospital groups, while the other suggested that the potential for genius is so often unrealized that high IQ scores actually measure little of concrete value and worth. Similarly, members of the citizen group did not believe that even extremely high IQ necessarily signaled a critical social resource. Said a woman, "I know some very bright people who don't contribute very much, who have a very difficult time. For me, they [persons with high and low IQ] may be equally dependent." Another agreed saying, to the amusement of others who knew her family, "I know. I mean, I lived with one [a person with high IQ] for fifteen years!"

At the other end of the scale, most participants argued that extremely low IQ scores would reflect a complex of individual and social deficits such that transplantation would be disallowed on other grounds. A person with an IQ of 30, for example, would have a series of other physical and psychosocial limitations that would not only make them marginal candidates medically but would be better measured by physical activity and social independence criteria. Members of the Down Syndrome Family Association group agreed that persons with extreme social and physical deficits would be better evaluated using criteria like physical activity, survival, and so forth, rather than IQ.

Here again there is independent verification of the groups' decisions. Following the fight over Sandra Jensen and Terry Urquart's candidacies, regulations were changed in both California and Calgary to permit the placement of persons with cognitive deficits on organ transplant waiting lists. Inspired by Jensen's fight for transplant eligibility, a bill prohibiting physicians and hospitals from denying access to life-saving transplantation based on the basis of a person's disability was passed by the California legislature in July 1996.[11] In Calgary, the debate over Terry Urquart's refusal resulted in a new standard recognizing family support as a value supporting the transplant candidacy of those with cognitive deficits. With these two cases, precedents were set in both Canada and the United States—acknowledging that however it is measured, "reasonable intelligence" does not serve as a sole independent criterion in transplant eligibility discussions.

Physical Activity

Criteria used to describe the medical need of patients on the transplant waiting list, usually defined as urgency status,[12] was inverted to create a category of "physical activity" in the hierarchy. Its importance was second only to "survival" as a criteria, reflecting a general belief that the "quality of life" as well as life itself is an important concern. And yet, as Figure 5.3 made clear, this was a contested criterion. It was far more highly valued by the first hospital group than by others, especially the Down

Figure 5.5
Physical Activity

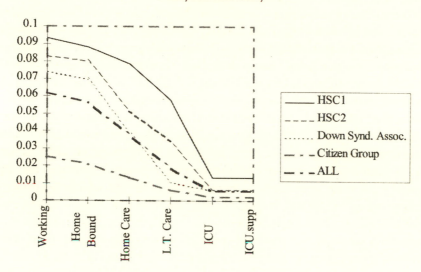

Syndrome Family Association participants. The question became at what level disabilities would be seen as barriers to transplantation.

Figure 5.5 graphically portrays the very consistent, level-2 judgments for this criterion. Given the small number of participating groups, the difference between ranking of "working" and "home bound" is insignificant. The former describes a person for whom a successful transplant will result in a wholly normal life with only minimal restrictions. The latter would be a person who, while limited in his or her physical range, needed little outside care and who would be expected to make a full recovery following a successful transplant.

Members of all groups agreed that persons requiring substantial continuing levels of care would be less suitable candidates. The reason was a belief that this level of disability would also entail a systemic fragility that might decrease the potential for survival. A quadriplegic was seen, for example, as more at risk in facing the rigors of organ transplant surgery than a neurologically normal person. Similarly, members of all groups largely dismissed as candidates persons requiring long-term, institutional assistance and certainly those who were in intensive care units. But in different groups a strong dissident voice argued that even extreme physical dependency should not be imposed as "quality of life" criteria prejudicing a person's candidacy.

Hospital staff members who work with physically challenged but mentally alert patients argued on the basis of their experience that a person with extreme physical limits may be as able, worthy, and valuable as any person. In discussing this criterion, members of most groups used as examples ALS patient Steven Hawking and quadriplegic actor Christopher Reeves. "If he needed a kidney or a liver, wouldn't you give it to him?" asked one person in the Citizens Group. Implicit was the idea that despite their physical limits, these people should be eligible for a transplant because their lives were not only public but also clearly full and worth living.

Across groups, the difficulty of discussing this criterion was twofold. While none wished to discriminate against those with physical limits, there was a reflexive assumption, challenged by some participants in each session, that increasing levels of physical impairment meant a necessarily decreasing quality of life. Further, most participants assumed that increasing levels of physical dependence would result in a decreasing ability to withstand the rigors of transplantation and posttransplant regimes. The first assumption was effectively countered in most discussions by reference to famous persons—for example, physicist Stephen Hawking—who have continued to work and contribute despite severe physical limitations. The latter assumption was one for which none of us had any data. A search of the literature after the sessions were concluded revealed data on the transplant survival rates of persons with limiting conditions. It may be that persons requiring even high levels of long-term support—quadriplegics like Christopher Reeve, for example—would be as likely to survive a transplant procedure as a person without his level of neurologic deficits. Thus, this stands as an important criterion in group decision making but one whose referents and supportive rationales were, in the end, unclear. As members of the Down syndrome group made clear, "disability" and its effect on both survival and life quality is a subjective, almost reflexive judgment that may not be supportable.

Social Independence

While members of all groups recognized the importance of social and familial support for persons facing a complex medical procedure requiring life-long postoperative medication, most saw this question as an "American" as opposed to a Canadian issue. "We've already decided [in Canada] that everyone deserves support," said a member of the hospital group.

"We may be in danger of losing the idea of that support," said a member of another session, "but we still have it, don't we?"

While all agreed the ideal candidate would be fully independent, requiring no extraordinary assistance after a successful transplant, all recognized that some would require greater familial and social assistance as a condition of long-term survival. That was seen by these Torontonians, however, as a natural right of citizenry and not as an element of extreme importance in candidate selection. Simply, it was assumed that all necessary home care and posttransplant support necessary would be provided to all patients. Thus, group members first defined and then devalued "insurer support," which in the United States refers to private medical insurance, as the use of provincial health services mandated to all citizens under the Canada Health Act.

For some, issues of social independence also referred to a level of fragility that might impact on survival. For others, familiar with the rigors of home and institutional care involving a patient's loved ones, however, extreme social dependence would be an issue were additional social support needed but not available. At this point members of several groups expressed their concern that increasing provincial and federal cuts in health care funding may make this an issue in future transplant eligibility discussions. A graduate student in social work who was training at the hospital said, in one group, that while less important now, diminished funding for hospital and health care would result in an environment where those without private means or private health insurance might be excluded as transplant candidates because of a lack of financial and other support.

In one hospital group this led to a brief discussion of the case of Benny Agrelo, a 15-year-old boy who received a liver transplant in the United States in 1994. Posttransplant he developed a reaction to medication that made him extremely ill. When he decided to cease taking his immunosuppressants, a court case was enjoined. The legal question was whether or not he could be forced to continue with his medications. The more general issues involved both his "quality of life" and the burden his treatment represented to his family. "It seems possible that Benny viewed his life as burdensome and costly for his mother and siblings," Michelle Oberman observed in a review of this case.[13]

While all agreed that independence is the optimal condition, most expressed a concern that family burden may be a factor or become a factor where social support is insufficient or unavailable. If home care and posttransplant care are generally available, then the importance of dependence can be minimized. This was, for example, the decision made in the Urquart case where family support was accepted as a substitute for individual ability as an indicator for the ability to understand and thus maintain posttransplant medication regimes. Should home support be unavailable, participants argued—or only available to those who can afford private care or insurance—then social dependence would become a more important criterion.

Thus, while social independence was not valued as a primary criteria, it was given moderate weight by most groups. The context of that decision is critical, however. It underscored the degree to which what may appear to be objective criteria in the end are based on social judgments or result from social contexts unrelated to the purely clinical needs of the patient.

Compliance

Real differences across groups resulted in discussions of patient compliance, defined in the literature and in focus group handouts as compliance with medical directives as a criterion in transplant eligibility decision making. This was clearly evident in Figure 5.3, where general consistency broke down over this criterion. Given its prevalence in the literature[14] and its general use at The Hospital for Sick Children, it was a shock when medical personnel in the first hospital group immediately distinguished between its use as a predictor of patient survival and one measuring social relations between patients and hospital staff. "Again and again it comes up" as an issue on the ward, one physician said, "and yet I have real problems with it." His concern, he continued, was that compliance is always a subjective judgment by staff about patient behavior and not necessarily a reliable predictor of posttransplant behavior.

"There are two ways it can be a problem," one doctor said. "One is because it alters your outcome, and makes your poor prognosis in terms of quality of life and life survival and survival length of that graft. And the other thing is the relationship we all treasure so much [with patients]. I think these are separate issues." Because they had already discussed survival as a criterion, members of this group then decided to define compliance as solely a measure of the relationship between the staff and the patient. Thus, failure to comply, group participants agreed, reflected on their ability to explain issues to the patients and not solely on a patient's adherence to medical directives.

Discussants thus spontaneously identified a technical problem called dilution occurring when a copy or near copy of an existing criterion is included in a hierarchy as if it were unique.[15] Dilution affects final results through the separate listing of what are, in effect, similar criteria, "diluting" the weight of one through the presentation of its duplicate parts. Not only is dilution a problem mathematically, but in this case it allows one apparently independent criterion ("compliance") to stand for one or more distinct criteria without making the relation between the two overt.

Members of the second hospital group were initially reluctant to accept the first group's lead. In a pretest questionnaire, members of this group ranked compliance as second only to survival as a transplant eligibility criteria. This was, they said in discussion, because it is used as a predictor of posttransplant survival. If it does not reflect that potential, they said, it obviously needed to be devalued. After a discussion of the literature in this area, researched after the first group's meeting, they accepted the first group, HSC1's definition. Still, most were somewhat shaken by the notion that patient compliance might not be a reliable predictor of posttransplant survival. This "changed everything," as one person pointed out, affecting the way all thought about compliance as a criterion in daily use at their hospital.

In passing, it is important to note how difficult it is to predict posttransplant performance on the basis of patient responses to preoperative behavior.[16] In a study of alcohol use by liver transplant recipients, for example, those with a history of alcohol abuse reported a lower rate of posttransplant drinking than did liver transplant recipients without a history of alcohol predictor of posttransplant patient activity.[17] More generally, some argue that "large numbers of patient do not comply with their prescribed treatment."[18] Daniel F. Chambliss, in a ten-year study of nursing practice at several hospitals, put the figure as high as 50 percent of patients as being at least periodically noncompliant.[19]

Participants in both the Down Syndrome Family Association and citizen discussion groups strongly emphasized compliance for wholly different reasons. For them, this was not a clinical but a social issue. For the former, compliance with medical directives was the "buy in" to appropriate treatment while the latter insisted that, in the end, "one has to trust the doctors to know what's best. "Buy in," participants explained, represented a measure of the patient's obligation to follow necessary pro-

cedures which, they assumed, would result in the best use of scarce transplant resources. Those in the citizen group agreed, although for them
compliance was also a measure of trust in the medical profession as well
as an indicator of social responsibility.

They argued that lay persons must assume that medical personnel don't
capriciously require activities that are nonsensical and that persons seeking rare organs and expensive social resources must trust their doctors.
"We don't know," one man said for all. "We have to trust they know
what they're doing." This did not mean, members of both groups continued, that a patient was obliged to accept all medical directives without
asking for an explanation. Each patient had a right to question medical
directives and to ask questions about them. Were those directives arbitrary, unsubstantiated—or even unexplained—members of these groups
said patients would not then be obliged to comply reflexively.

Four different responses were received, therefore, based on four distinct
interpretations of what "compliance" signified despite the fact that all
received the same preparatory materials, including definitions of all criteria to be used in discussion. It was the heavy emphasis on compliance
by the citizen group that skewed its final judgments, contributing to a
higher than acceptable inconsistency index.

These different perspectives masked a general agreement when issues
of social and medical values were clarified. All participants agreed that
in cases where a patient's behavior clearly would jeopardize a graft organ
donation—for example, a continual refusal to take oral medication—that
noncompliance should mean noncandidacy. It is also, however, a measure
of social rather than clinical values in staff-patient relationships.

An example used in one discussion serves to make the distinction clear.
Consider a potential organ recipient who takes her prescribed medications but who also uses Chinese medicinal teas purchased for her by concerned parents and friends. A staff member insists that use of those
traditional teas be stopped. There is, however, no evidence that they will
in any way affect the efficacy of prescription medications. While staff
might not like patients to use traditional remedies, labeling this patient
"noncompliant"—and thus denying candidacy—would reflect not patient suitability but staff prejudices.

In a hospital report based on this work, compliance therefore was split
into two distinct criteria. Where it related to long-term survival, it was
included as a subset of that criteria rather than an independent variable.
As an independent criterion, however, it was used to define staff-patient
relationships. In this construction, compliance is dependent on patient

understanding and acceptance of directives explained and justified to them by hospital staff. Its importance rests solely on those activities that can be shown clearly to impact on patient fitness for a transplant procedure and the potential for posttransplant survival.

By separating compliance into two distinct criteria in this manner, one solely based on patient behavior and another reflecting staff-patient relations, the apparently disparate views of these diverse groups were reconciled. The critical issue was not, in the end, ignorance of transplant protocols by nonprofessionals (Down syndrome and citizen groups) but a complex of social and clinical definitions masquerading as a single, supposedly well-defined, criterion.

DISCUSSION

The advantages of asking diverse focus groups to evaluate a hierarchy prepared from a literature review rather than one they generated are now clear. First, there is a saving of time. It took an average of two months to set up each hospital meeting, to coordinate the hectic schedules of staff persons involved in patient care, administration, consultation, and other responsibilities. Were each group to generate its own hierarchy, then to regularize those hierarchies before beginning an evaluation, would have been simply too time consuming for an experimental pilot program like this one. Even were it possible, however, the resulting criteria set would have lacked a single attribute of the one generated by the approach adopted here. A literature-based hierarchy permitted members of various groups to consider a single criteria list whose individual parts were independently validated. Thus, literature-based answers to questions about specific issues, either their general use in other settings or the data surrounding their utility, was close at hand. Finally, this approach offered a mechanism by which generally accepted criteria could be evaluated.

Unexpectedly, use of a literature-based hierarchy permitted a critique of both generally accepted criteria and the underlying values that support them. Because many hospital participants had studied the literature, discussion of this hierarchy required they see its assumptions within the context of their own daily experience. This is a benefit not to be underestimated. Confusions of sign and signifier, of clinical and social values, occur again and again in bioethics as in other areas of ethical dispute. As Margaret A. Somerville says, "These confusions span, first, the domain of semantics—confusion in definition; confusion created through choice of language; and confusion of association and analogy. Second, they span important areas of ethical and legal analysis."[20] To the degree that literature is the basis for professional opinions or policies, confusion must reign there too. This is what the discussions revealed to many hospital-based participants.

Naturally and without direction, group discussion focused on these confusions, seeking data to support or reject one or another definition, identifying values previously hidden. IQ tests don't measure intelligence but a type of intelligence that while important is not sufficient in and of itself to determine life and death issues; nor is it the sole predictive measure of an individual's ability and willingness to follow posttransplant regimes. Its use is pragmatic—"It's a firm number"—and a value emphasizing one type of intelligence over another. Similarly, compliance is a widely used value whose utility as a predictor is uncertain. But it is also a critical value within the hospital culture,[21] one whose social importance may outweigh its predictive function. These divisions and confusion were made clear in discussion.

Finally, the advantage of using a broad set of participants in sequential, group-specific focus groups is now obvious. The hospital, involved stake-holders, and the general public can all have different perceptions of the issues surrounding a specific dilemma. Within both the hospital and the community it serves, persons may discuss what appears to be the same criterion (compliance, intelligence, survivability, and so forth) but do so with very different interpretations of not just the relevance but the meaning of the criterion itself. Think of these differences as problems of translation between the languages of various constituent groups. Until these differences can be identified and the languages used in debate brought into accord, the potential for litigious disagreement and public confrontation is real. That was one lesson learned from the disputed cases outlined in the previous chapter. Involving representatives of these groups in the process critiques the official hierarchy while identifying specific points of consensus and disagreement. It permits the views of diverse perspectives to be combined and coordinated.

REFLECTIONS

To date, perhaps the greatest practical benefit of this work has been educational. Members of citizen and Down syndrome discussion groups were first surprised and then chastened by the difficult balancing act these judgments required. "This is hard!" members of both groups said at their respective meetings. "I'm glad I don't have to do this for real!" said someone in the citizen group. In postsession discussions, participants said the exercise gave them new understanding and new respect for the difficult choices attending physicians and hospital staff must make in this area.

For their part, hospital personnel found it useful and sometimes humbling to compare and listen to their colleagues. Because all members of the group had their opinions solicited, persons who are often not heard in clinical rounds—nurses, for example—or who are heard as less than equal voices (social workers, bioethicists) were given full participation. In expressing their views, each participant had to consider his or her value set and distinguish it from what might otherwise seem to be a purely clinical judgment. "It's one thing to have values," said a participant in the first hospital group. "It's another thing to have to express them and still something else to have to defend them!" The degree to which many of their judgments were value based and not solely clinical was for some a chastening revelation.

One goal of this program at the hospital was to determine whether or not the MCDM approach could forge a unified view that might serve as the basis for a policy statement. These results answered that question affirmatively. Utilizing them effectively has been a subject of some discussion, however. At present, hospital policy must result from broad and extensive consultation with clear and numerically consistent results. This typically requires survey-based examinations of broad sample populations. It is neither economically practical nor practically feasible to hold twenty or thirty focus groups, however. Neither the funding nor the will for this type of time-consuming process is presently available in the financially restricted context of Ontarian hospital-based medicine.

Data from this study was first transformed into a "patient information brochure" designed to explain to perspective transplant patients and their families both the rights and obligations of transplant candidacy. It was seen by administrators, however, as lacking the type of qualitative numerical support required of official policy. The results of these focus groups is therefore being reformulated as a draft policy statement to be submitted, with an explanation of its methodology, to hospital and community groups. When completed and approved by research committees, this document will present the focus groups' determinations in a manner that can be subjected to a broad sampling of hospital and client-based personnel.

Thus, this work leads, at present, to the type of policy statement that can be examined using more traditional survey methods. That work is in progress.

In terms of the broader issues this book addresses, however, tentative conclusions can be offered. Consensus is possible even where differences of definition and perspective exist. Further, it can be achieved without the impetus of expensive legal fights or damaging public controversy. Neither truths nor hard and fast clinical rules are returned in this process, however. Guidelines that are social and clinical at once are its logical result. As the participants in this program were quick to point out, their judgments may not serve in extraordinary cases. While most believe severe physical limitations and social dependency are an at least modest counterindication for transplant candidates, all recognized the possibility of exceptions. None would deny Stephen Hawking the opportunity for prolonged life despite the limits imposed on his life by Lou Gehrig's disease, for example.

Persons in the Down Syndrome Family Association group wished to make an exception to their denial of IQ's value as a criteria by insisting those with "real genius" be given preferential treatment. For them, and for others in these groups, society's needs for the exceptional may outweigh general concerns for consistency and equal treatment. Thus, all recognized that what was offered in this exercise was a general perspective that should inform decision making at the individual level, not a substitute for the case-by-case judgments that are made every day in this and other hospitals.

Further, consensus demands first and foremost agreement at the level of definition, not reflexive adherence to a general principle. Each group interpreted the definitions in the handouts in light of their own experiences, values, and social positions. Within the context of the hospital groups, people discovered assumptions made on the basis of that experience often conflicted with other, deeper perceptions. It is not knowledge alone, the amount of data one has acquired, but knowledge within the context of social, cultural, and personal perspectives that will inhibit or facilitate agreement in contentious areas of debate.

Finally, consensus and the definitions that permit it occurs at a specific scale. They occur within national, regional, and community boundaries; within the context of national, regional, and cultural values. The Canadian imperative to universally switch to treatment noted in these groups would not necessarily be operative in a U.S. study. Still, as a general rule one may say that the more precise a model's definitions, the more useful its conclusions will be at the scale it was administered. Even where consensus is reached, however, it will not serve to wholly resolve the practical and complex decisions a clinician, politician, or average citizen must make for or with a fragile person whose individual perspective will be based on a complex of specific needs, family context, and personal history. What these judgments present, in the end, is a socially cohesive background to support and ground decisions affecting the individual within his or her community.

6

Humanness, Personhood, and the Fragile

INTRODUCTION

In denying a hospital's request for permission to discontinue ventilator support for Baby K, a severely anencephalic child, Virginia District Court judge Mr. Clyde Hilton ruled in 1993 that, "Just as an AIDS patient seeking ear surgery is 'otherwise qualified' to receive treatment despite poor long-term prospects for living, Baby K is 'otherwise qualified' to receive ventilator treatment."[1] Individuals deserve equal care, in other words, irrespective of the deficits they may suffer or the prognosis they may face. Anencephaly is a rare condition occurring in early pregnancy that results in the failure of the brain—but not the brain stem—to develop. In this and another, well-known case, In re T.A.C.P.,[2] it was held that failure to treat the anencephalic—and by extension the PVS (permanent vegetative state) patient—would create an unacceptable category of living but unequal individuals, a set of nonpersons burdened with a set of diminished human rights.

A vast, critical literature has grown up around these and similar decisions.[3] Ethicists, bioethicists, and physicians have questioned the insistence that all living humans, whatever their clinical condition, must be perceived as equally entitled to treatment under the law. Either on the basis of "quality of life" standards, or from the perspective of "futility" judgments, many have argued that the law's traditional standard reflects neither the values of society nor the realities of contemporary medical practice.[4] On the one hand, therefore, there, is the insistence that all are equal under the law irrespective of physical or cognitive limits. On the other, there is a professional literature—often supported by popular sentiment—saying some individuals are so frail, so disabled, and with lives so short as to exist outside the otherwise universal protection otherwise offered all living human beings.

At the heart of this difference is the distance between a medical model's focus on a patient's clinical condition, his or her physical divergence from the population's norm, and the legal system's insistence on equality of persons irrespective of their individual deficits. The former is defined by observable difference, by "a hidden negative assumption that what is important about a person is his or her injury, disease, deficiency, problem, need, empty half."[5] The latter is driven by an insistence that no distinction be made between human beings who are assumed to be equally vested with an identical packet of legal, moral, and social rights irrespective of their physical, social, or economic status.[6] Whatever their level of physical dependence or cognitive dysfunction, however great or small their degree of social contribution, every individual is guaranteed the opportunity to equal treatment.[7]

While often defined in terms of anencephaly, the issues extend far beyond this specific problem. Should one ventilate and otherwise maintain all those infants whose life expectancy is minimal and whose physical deficits are equally or more severe? There are other genetic conditions—for example, trisomy 18—that similarly result in severe retardation, physical deformities, and diminished life expectancy in infants. At the other end of the scale, the issue is often posed in terms of adult patients in a permanent vegetative state, those who have at least some surviving autonomic functions but who by reason of stroke, traumatic injury, or degenerative illness have lost the capacities of perception and reason. Should they be maintained through the technologies of mechanical life support? Do we accept them as persons, despite their deficits, and more fundamentally, do we accept their humanity as similar to our own?

Here we have another paradoxical problem of definition. Where is the line between those we treat and those we do not? When is it senseless to maintain a patient through mechanical means, and when is it a worthy action and goal? Some would decide these questions on the basis of "outcome assessment," evaluation based on the probability of a successful outcome of one or another clinical procedure. But is stabilizing the anencephalic infant a successful outcome, or a futile gesture? What about a patient with ALS or MS? At what point does continuation itself become an undesirable goal? Put another way, at what stage of disability is a life so bounded and restricted as to be no life at all?

The bioethical literature general advances a position distinguishing between the sentient (or in the case of infants, the potentially sentient) individual and those whose cognitive faculties are nonexistent. "It is only to persons with capacity to value existence that respect is owed," John Harris said, echoing a common viewpoint in his book, *The Value of Life*.[8] The anencephalic—or the patient in a permanent vegetative state—can't value his or her own existence and so, it would follow, we need not. And yet, As Judith F. Daar points out, "To date, in early every known case in which the patient [or the patient's family] has sought treatment and the doctors have objected on the grounds that treatment offers no medical benefit, courts have found in favor of the patient."[9] If there was social unanimity on nontreatment in cases of extreme limitation, the problem might be more easily resolved. As Hanley noted in her analysis of *In re T.A.C.P.*, "The case might have been decided differently had T.A.C.P.'s parents shown there was a 'consensus' in society to redefine anencephaly as death, or to approach the harvesting of organs from infants with anencephaly as if they were dead."[10] But just as a public general agreement on abortion has failed, so, too, has there been none in this area. The courts have insisted upon a "life interest," on traditional values of human life's sanctity despite the assertions of the majority of authors writing in the bioethical literature.

MODELING

The question arising from the decision known as *In re Baby K* is clear, if stark: How do we distinguish between the HIV+ adult and the anencephalic infant without denying the humanity and the personhood of either? Are those differences fundamental or merely clinically descriptive? More generally, the issue is the distinctions we may perceive but cannot easily express between "normal" adults or children and the fragile of different age groups and with different cognitive abilities.

These questions might have been addressed through focusing a hierarchy or discussion group using a social choice procedure model to define a single treatment alternative for patients with extreme deficits. In such a model, the goal would be "levels of treatment" and alternatives would be: no care (no hydration or nutrition), palliative care (keep them comfortable), stabilizing care (ventilation for the anencephalic), full care (maximizing health potential), and extreme care (organ transplantation, for example). These could then be applied to a variety of problematic alternatives: adults in a permanent vegetative state, infants with anencephaly, those with degenerative neurologic disorders (ALS, fulminating MS, etc.), or other conditions.

But that would beg the primary issue considered by the courts and by some bioethicists: Are the lives of those with extreme deficits so different as to exclude a "duty to care" by professionals? Where is society's obligation, and how do we define it? To begin with "levels of treatment" would encourage the assumption that in a context of scarcity, of declining monies for health care, that choices must be made. But if we decide no distinctions can be made on the basis of these criteria without denying some human persons on the basis of disability alone, that construct would be moot. The question addressed in this study was the more fundamental problem of humanness, on whether or not we believe extreme deficits or an inevitably foreshortened life diminishes the patient's status as an equal member of our community, one equally deserving of our care.

For this reason, focus groups were asked to discuss a social welfare function model describing criteria defining "humanness." Treatment alternatives may be assumed, based on the model, but its goal is to define the relative strength of the criteria contributing to a definition of humanness, not to match clinical procedure with social assessment. In contemporary bioethics, many treat humanness and personhood as synonyms, while others insist "personhood" is the critical criterion for bioethical consideration.[11] Humanness was chosen because in the longer debate of eugenics, and of life boat ethics, the concept seemed more central, with "personhood" a subset of the more general category of humanness. As background, members of both groups were given a brief description of several critical cases—*In the Matter of Baby K, In re T.A.C.P,* and so forth—and of the issues they represented.

Constructing a hierarchy to address these problems was facilitated by the literatures on both personhood and humanness. Joseph Fletcher's well-known essay on humanhood was selected as a convenient starting point for a discussion of what we mean—socially, clinically, and biologically—when we talk about ourselves as members of a species.[12] Modifications have been made, however, both to facilitate modeling and to acknowledge the work of others in this area.

Defining Humanness

The following criteria were used to define the class of humanhood and its subset, personhood:

1. *Physical Signature:*

1a. Genetic makeup: Humanness includes conformity to a species-specific genetic pattern dictating a set of innate mental and physical potentials that are typically realized over time, usually through social instruction (children) and interaction (adults). Humans are also genetically gifted, "hard-wired" in the current jargon, with an innate potential for learning both tool use and language,[13] the latter making possible (3a) communication, abstract thought, and (4a) demonstrable self-awareness.

1b. Physical form (gross): The human form is defined by limbs allowing bipedal movement, arms with hands whose opposing fingers allow grasping and manipulation, external sensors (eyes, ears, etc.) and speech organs, and other characteristic morphological attributes.

1c. Physical appearance: Departure from socially accepted standards of external appearance, irrespective of gross physical form, may result in social prejudice such that people feel "unhuman." The history of adverse treatment on the basis of skin color, or departure from social standards of appearance, demands the inclusion of this criterion, as does the psychological literature on children with obvious disabilities or visible deformities.[14]

2. *Cognitive Signature:*

Approximately a third of Fletcher's criteria are directly or indirectly concerned with mental functioning and capability including: "neocortical function," "self-awareness," and "time sense." For convenience, these are combined into three attributes:

2a. "Intelligence" here refers to higher brain functions of categorization, organization, storage, and integration of data. Several of Fletcher's criteria (for example, "time sense") are subsumed in this category. He discussed IQ as a general measure of this criteria, and we note in passing that while there are difficulties with that measure it remains in general use.

2b. "Perception" describes preintegrative neurologic response to sensation and stimuli irrespective of mediating organization or categorization.

2c. "Autonomic functions" are primary reflexes, including respiration, sucking, grasping, and the like. The relation of autonomic "brain stem" functions to questions of patient "life," and thus patient humanity, has been well reviewed.[15]

3. *Communal Signature:*

Almost 50 percent of Fletcher's list is partly or wholly concerned with the interpersonal and social characteristics of humanness.

3a. Communicative potential: Whatever a person's social or interpersonal potential, it requires the ability to communicate before it can be realized. A greater or lesser communicative ability is a prerequisite for other elements in this signature.

3b-c. Social capacity: "A person exists not in isolation from others, but only through relationships. We are as we relate."[16] Individual potentials are activated only through social association, defined here, after Fletcher, as the capacity to (3b) relate to others and to (3c) care for others. A psychopath may have excellent relational skills, for example, but be unable to "care" for others or consider their needs.

3d. Attachments: The ability to form sustaining relations with others is an essential human element. Failure of short-term memory or integrative function in patients with conditions like Korsokov's syndrome or Alzheimer's disease, or resulting from trauma to the brain, may result in an inability to form or in some cases to maintain sustaining attachments.[17]

3e. Humans also are marked by what Lewis Thomas called a "drive to be useful," materially and socially, to their fellow species members.[18] The drive to be useful may be understood as a drive for self-meaning through public acts and service.

4. *Individual Signature:*

Whatever their physical condition, intellectual ability, or social station, all humans have individual experiences, relations, and qualities. If they can be stored and processed (2a), then according to Fletcher's paradigm they will typically result in:

4a. Self-awareness, the end result of cognitive potential, social training, and communicative capacity.

4b. Self-control, which is similarly the result of social training and unimpaired cognitive functioning.

4c. Creativity, which while not an element in Fletcher's paradigm, is so honored by society at large, as to warrant inclusion here.

4d. Uniqueness: Each person's history reveals a series of decisions, of associations and accomplishments, which over time become a personalized signature. 3b allows for those choices to be recognized.

Figure 6.1
Degree of Humanness

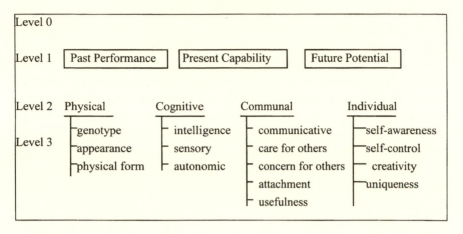

5. *Time:*

Humans share a singular and complex time sense composed of memory (of prior events), hopes and plans (future events), and immediate realities (the present).[19] Further, humans develop capacities and abilities over time and may lose some or all of those capacities and abilities at any time as a result of illness or injury.

The hierarchy based on this model is presented in Figure 6.1.

Focus Groups

The hierarchy's inclusion of interpersonal as well as individual attributes is in line with both the perspectives presented by the organ transplant focus groups and with current thinking on the interrelated and social nature of our species.[20] Using temporal categories—past achievement, current performance, and future potential—as level-1 attributes addresses not merely the potential longevity or demonstrable history but also the broad social context of that candidate. By considering temporality as an organizing level-1 concern, outcome assessment (futurity) is addressed within what is necessarily a broader temporal and social context. Answers to this formulation also may serve as a critique of a parallel literature in gerontology that argues either for or against weighing a person's past achievements as well as his or her future potential in the allocation of health care resources.[21]

Some might argue that genetic characteristics should be included as a level-2 criteria, that there are essential genes that allow one to exist and be human. Unless genetic make-up is raised in the hierarchy—or at least a criteria emphasizing "defining" genes as opposed to those governing pigmentation, sex, hair color, and so forth—the potential is left open for certain animals species and the androids of science fiction to claim equal status in our society. As chapter 2 made clear, however, others use the argument of genetic similarity to insist upon the protected status of higher primates. It was placed as a level-3 criterion in an attempt to determine its importance to participants, to assess the degree to which members would argue for its inclusion at a higher level, or perhaps, for its devaluation in the hierarchy as a whole. While contentious, the ramifications of the decision to include it here are discussed both in this chapter and in the next on the basis of participant responses.

Framed in this manner, the question becomes one involving not only allocation of scarce resources—who do we treat?—but more important, one of definition in the context of a higher order principle. Who do we accept within the protected sphere of sanctified human life; how do we define what we mean by "us," both medically and socially? To address these questions, two focus groups were constituted in The Hospital for Sick Children, Toronto, pilot program. The first involved a heterogeneous group of eight staff persons from the hospital: staff psychiatrists, social workers, bioethicists, neonatologists, pediatricians, and pastoral counselors. The second group included seven persons from the Toronto Beaches community, a citizen "control" group whose members were not expert in the issue but interested in the general problems health care presents to society at large. One woman in the group, a landscape architect, was the mother of an anencephalic infant who had died more than a decade previously.

It took both groups approximately four hours to complete their evaluation of the model. For members of the citizens group, whose members had to return to their families, or to work, and for those in the hospital group whose participation pulled them from their duties, this was a marathon session. Indeed, hospital participants broke their discussion into two sessions because it was impossible to find a single, four-hour block that would free all for this exercise. To maintain the continuity of discussion and shorten the procedure where possible, evaluation of level-3 criteria was completed for one time frame rather than repeated for each separate level-1 criterion. Level-3 assessments for both groups were then

Figure 6.2
Level-1 Criteria

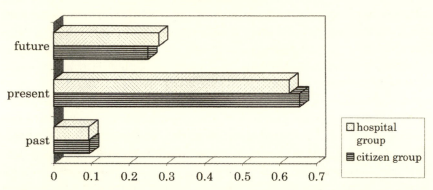

copied to the other time frames. The rest of this chapter summarizes these results, interpreting them in the context of the broader qualitative discussion.

LEVEL-1 CRITERIA

In the pairwise comparisons of level-1 criteria (see Figure 6.2), both groups almost equally emphasized the present condition over past performance and future potential. This reflected, first and foremost, a general belief in the individual human life as distinct, remarkable, and precious. "I think that as a human being there has to be a general value that we hold true to across the board whether it's babies or old people or anyone," said one woman to general agreement. Irrespective of physical condition, past performance, or future potential, she argued, that humanhood demands recognition. In their discussion, members of the medical group agreed. "I think everybody is religious that way, that there is something special about being human," said one pediatrician. For members of these communities there is a presumption of humanity (and of human personhood) whose individual characteristics may be unclear but whose importance is not. At any moment and in any context, its denial requires strong and incontrovertible evidence.

Among the citizen discussants, the present was described as defining a concrete reality against an "iffy" future. Simply, the future is too uncertain to allow for its dominance in this discussion, they agreed. But because all believed the future of an individual is of importance to society at large,

futurity's potential weighed more heavily than an individual's past performance. When asked whether a history of social involvement and contribution might not define a person's humanity—the Japanese view that
one spends a lifetime becoming truly human—members of both groups
demurred.

In this discussion members of both groups grappled with how to take
what was, to them, an abstract idea—humanness or personhood—and
make it concrete. While hospital group members often did this in terms
of specific diagnoses and conditions, those in the citizen group used more
general situations. In discussing temporality, for example, a forty-three-
year-old high school teacher in fact argued against valuing past performance with an organ transplant analogy. In comparing himself to an
infant—"If there was only one liver and we both needed it to live"—he
said that in choosing between them, he'd argue for the infant. "He's saying
he's had 43 years," another discussant summarized. [If a choice had to be
made], he'd like that four-year old to have the same chance he's had."
Others agreed, using a type of "fair innings" argument to devalue past
performance in its comparisons with future potential and present condition.[22]

Devaluing past history was expected among hospital staff members.
After all, each had chosen a pediatric specialty and children have no long
personal history of achievement. How a five-or even a fifteen-year old
will turn out in twenty years is simply unknowable. Whatever their "past,"
it is likely an insufficient guide to future potential. As a neonatologist
explained, "I have to make decisions, but I would hate to do that based
on a six-year-old's past performance." Others agreed. "Are we going to
decide [his future] on [the basis of] Johnny's finger painting? Or Margaret's
ability at doing sums?"

More generally, however, members of the hospital group believed that
near term future potential may be a clinical determinant in extreme cases.
"If I'm oblivious to the future," said one participant, a neonatologist, "I'd
have to ventilate the trisomy 18 infant. The life expectancy is a week, or
in five percent of the cases, perhaps beyond a month. Obviously, I think
that would be inappropriate." Also known as Edward's syndrome, trisomy
18 is a genetic disorder resulting in severe mental retardation and multiple
physical deformities. While Edward's syndrome infants have a developed
cerebral cortex, they share with anencephalics the label of futility, of a
chronic and severely limiting condition that will be terminal within
months or a year.

If ventilating a trisomy 18 infant—or an anencephalic—is "inappropriate," how did the hospital group perceive treatment of adults with similarly foreshortened life spans and cognitive deficits? Like participants in the citizen discussion group, members of the hospital group did not assume that the elderly should receive special treatment because of their long social histories and rich interpersonal pasts. Those whose future is truncated by severe stroke, Alzheimer's disease, or other disorders that might deprive them of future abilities should not, a member said, be valued simply on the basis of past performance. Indeed, as one doctor said dismissively, it would be like offering an organ transplant to an eighty-year-old person. While all agreed present condition and need outweigh all other time frames, most also were inclined to offer futurity as a criterion over past achievement in their deliberations.

Members of the citizen group did note one exception. A history of extreme antisocial acts affects determination of a person's humanity in the present. Here the discussion centered on Canadian serial killer, Clifford Olsen, and what most saw as his diminished humanity. Just as a history of violence against others was seen as a counterindication in organ transplant eligibility discussions, so, too, was it a factor in this discussion. "Inhuman acts define inhumanity," as one participant put it and thus diminish an individual's claim to humanity's membership and the common weal.

This perspective is one that has been heard repeatedly by courts considering the punishment of those convicted of vicious crimes. In 1993, the Liverpool, England, trial judge sentencing two ten-year-old boys for the brutal murder of toddler James Bulger, for example, called the preadolescent killers "monsters" and inhuman. In sentencing Yigal Amir for the political assassination of Israeli Prime Minister Yitzhak Rabin, for example, Chief Judge Edmond Levy, said of Amir that, "He does not merit any regard whatsoever, except pity, because he has lost his humanity."[23] More recently, it was expressed as justification for the sentence given to Timothy McVeigh after he was convicted of the bombing of the U.S. Federal building in Oklahoma City. "When Timothy McVeigh made the decision to murder, maim, and destroy all these people," a survivor told reporters, "he gave up the right to be called a human being."[24]

Members of these groups thus perceived humanness as a birthright, like citizenship, one assumed unless somehow disavowed by conscious action. It is incorrect to assume a person is less-than-human or a nonperson solely because of a foreshortened future, they argued. Similarly, humanness does not accrue on the basis of past performance. It is defined instead by one's current condition, a person's present actions and needs. While care is to

Figure 6.3
Level-2 Criteria

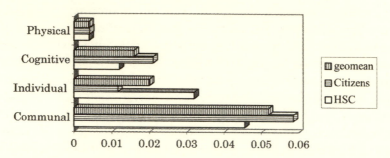

be extended to all within the human circle, inhuman acts against others may be used in extreme and rare cases to deny an individual's claim to common care and protection. Discussions of level-2 criteria refined what participants perceived as the boundaries of that protective circle.

LEVEL-2 CRITERIA

At the second level, Figure 6.3, communal attributes—those defining social and interpersonal abilities—dominated the judgments of both groups. The geometric mean of both groups is included here as an indicator of a shared, communal position. Similarly, both devalued physically defining characteristics (physical appearance, gross physical form, genetic make-up), while disagreeing on the attribute sets comparing criteria sets defining individual and cognitive elements. In reviewing these judgments—and their relation to both the idea and ideal of humanness as well as to clinical judgments—it is easiest to start with the least valued criterion and work forward to those that were more strongly valued.

Physical Characteristics

There was intense discussion in the hospital discussion group over the importance of physical characteristics, both those that may bear upon the appearance of the individual—"It has such an effect on the 'quality of life'—and more generally on the place of genetic differences in defining who will and will not be protected within the sanctity of human life syndrome. A psychiatrist specializing in facial deformities was queried

about her view of the importance of social ostracism resulting from physical malformations. This was, one suggested, a matter of "quality of life"
rather than of humanness itself. Still, continued another, social prejudice
based on physical difference may effectively set one person apart from his
or her contemporaries, effectively challenging a person's common membership on the basis of prejudice alone. Was this something they wanted
to endorse?

To the surprise of many group members, a bioethicist then commented
that a significant problem faced by genetic counselors at the hospital was
the desire of some parents to abort a fetus where amniocentesis showed
a developing infant with cleft palate and harelip but without other serious
deficits. The idea of a newborn who looked different, even if that difference would be correctable, was harder for some expectant parents than
an otherwise normal looking child with spinal bifida, for example. Genetic counselors at the hospital found it difficult when correctable facial
malformations were seen, by clients, as a reason to terminate a pregnancy.
Members of this discussion group were adamant that while parents had
the right to decide on abortion in Canada, that denying life on the basis
of atypical appearance—especially that which can later be surgically cor-
rected—was wrong. One physician summed up the group's sentiment
when he said flatly, "No physical state should be a deterrent as long as
they're [claimants] cognitively normal."

Citizen group participants reached similar conclusions. In the system
of pairwise comparisons, the devaluation of physical characteristics was
obvious. It was not that physical qualities were perceived as unimpor-
tant—"of course they're terribly important. We're all embodied," said one
woman—but rather that their importance is less important in defining
the essence of humanhood. In explaining the difference he perceived
between physical and cognitive attributes, for example, one group member asked another: "Which is more important? That your body works, or
your brain works? Is it more important that you think or that you are?"
In comparing social and physical attributes, another person put the question with equal bluntness: "Don't you see this difference: The person
looks human but acts inhuman. Or, the person looks different but acts
very human?"

At the next level of analysis, members of both groups valued genetic
make-up as twice as important as either measure of physical appearance.
Members of the medical group did this "Not just for itself," as one participant explained, "but because it determines so many other [individual]
characteristics." But it retained a low overall value in the model because,

as another insisted, what is important is not the limits imposed by birth but the life that is lived by the person him- or herself. Within the citizen group, genetics was assumed to be somewhat more important but none were able to explain its importance to them. "We're learning so much," said one. The general feeling was that increasingly genetic knowledge will affect the physical self—and states of wellness or illness—but that "humanness" and personhood are something different. In this context they discussed the potential human of "thinking machines," using television and movie models as examples of how nongenetically based beings still might be "human." In this discussion one used the android Mr. Data, a character on the TV show "Star Trek: The Next Generation," and another remembered the computer personality "Hal" in the movie *2001*.

Unlike members of the hospital discussion group, members of this group generally lacked practical experience with persons at the boundaries of either physical or behavioral limits. They recognized this lack. Like members of the citizen organ transplant eligibility group, they believed that in some areas they had to trust the physicians and nurses whose practical expertise extended beyond their own. They found in science fiction a metaphor for the problem of cybernetics, of the potential of beings with cognitive and social abilities but without the genetic and biological history we reflexively think of as "human." This is not a trivial way to address these issues. As Oliver Sacks points out, some autistic persons take the android Mr. Data—his self-conscious if sometimes fumbling attempts to mimic human behavior rules—as a mirror of their own frustrations and limits.[25] At another level, science fiction writers like Isaac Asimov have, for more than thirty years, used the android or the robot as tools with which to explore what we mean by humanness, personhood, and their attendant rights and responsibilities.[26]

Cognition

The citizen group judged cognition (higher order cerebral functions, perceptual functions, autonomic functions) to be a more important criterion set than the complex labeled "individual characteristics," a set valued over cognitive criteria by hospital participants. For all, cognition permitted by higher order cerebral functioning defined the potential for the development of individual characteristics while hospital personnel saw attributes of individuality (self-control, self-awareness, etc.) as a more primary concern.

The importance of perceptual limits and autonomic functions were strongly devalued by both groups. In both sessions, one or another participant independently used Helen Keller as an example of a person with severe perceptual deficits whose humanity and personhood was unquestioned. Persons with diseases affecting autonomic functions like respiration, for example, ALS patients like Stephen Hawking, and spinal injury patients like Superman actor Christopher Reeve, also were discussed in an attempt to understand the relation between human personhood to be preserved and specific deficit. With each example, the humanness of the person with a critical limit was underscored, for discussants, by his or her respective social or intellectual contribution to society as a whole. Enormously severe deficits may be overcome, all agreed, without affecting what one physician called the "spark" of humanness that he sought and treasured. "I have worked with two kids who were born without any function below the neck and they have done fine," added a psychiatrist in the group. "But then, they were extremely bright."

For both groups, "cognition" was the critical defining criteria in this category. But diminished cognitive function did not necessarily result in diminished humanity, both groups agreed. Here the discussion centered on children with cognitive deficits—for example, persons with Down syndrome. The neonatologist used the "six-year-old who is a 'special child' who is accepted and contented in the family, the Down Syndrome child" as an example of one whose cognitive limits, defined genetically, should not exclude that person from care, treatment, and the support we give all other human persons.

Members of both groups thus would disagree with pediatricians who have advised parents to not permit corrective life-saving surgery for infants with Down syndrome, for example Baby Doe[27] or Baby Ross.[28] The potential "quality of life" of such an infant is based, participants said, not solely on limits defined clinically but also on a broad complex of social, familial, and intergenerational factors. None doubted the importance of cognitive deficits. All agreed, however, that the essential issue defining the humanity of the individual lies not in individual attributes or cognitive limits alone, but in the degree of participation in or alienation from the set of communal attributes defining interpersonal characteristics.

In the citizen group as well, the value and importance of those with cognitive limits was expressed in terms of persons with Down syndrome. "They're so loving," said one person. "They're important for their openness." In this group, the complete absence of higher brain function did raise fundamental questions, however. One man, whose father was in a coma for three weeks following a stroke, raised this issue. "That was not my father," he told the group. "That was not a person any more. He was just a body because he was gone. Now, he came back. But my mother, my brothers, and I were prepared for him to not be that person [we knew] because [in the coma] there was absolutely no response." Thus, for him, the complete and sustained absence of higher brain function would deny the personhood of the individual, the "spark" of humanity we seek in each person. For this man and his family, who their father had been (past performance) did not serve to consecrate the body of the patient in a coma. For them, the issue was his immediate condition and the potential of his "returning," of awakening.

While all understood his concerns, not everyone agreed with him. Here there were indeed two camps. A woman whose husband had died of cancer and whose father had died of Alzheimer's disease agreed wholeheartedly. The idea of lingering without consciousness or in the shadow of declining abilities was, to her, intolerable. But the woman who had given birth to a short-lived, anencephalic child disagreed. Understanding their concerns and fears, she held to a belief that that humanness, and perhaps personhood, may still reside even within the context of extremely severe limits.

Individual and Communal

Recognizing communal over all other criteria sets was, for some hospital personnel, a recognition of their personal as well as clinical involvement with the fragile patient. "I have a hard time removing myself from the situation," admitted one pastoral counselor. "Maybe it's the phenomonologist in me. I have a shared meaning with this . . . entity. I can't remove myself." And so to the extent that she feels a tie to the severely limited patient—and to that person's family who requires her counseling—the restricted patient gains humanity and personhood as a result.

More generally, all agreed that the decision to treat and care for fragile patients often reflects not simply a clinical judgment but, more important, the relationship between the patient and those who love and care for them. As John Hardwig wrote several years ago, "There is no way to detach the lives of patients from the lives of those who are close to them."[29] The status of the severely limited patient is weighed by members of this group not in a social vacuum but in the context of a complex of interpersonal relationships that includes family members, clinical caregivers, and society at large. This is the reality of clinical decision making, as the medical discussion group's neonatologist explained. "The parent who brings in a child with severe CP [cerebral palsy], who has had repeated admissions, and has aspirated one more time. The parent says, 'I know when she's in pain. I know when she's unhappy.' But no one else is party to that language. Why do we keep on doing what we're doing? It's the subjectivity of this [parental] interaction."

In defining level-3 criteria Lewis Thomas' "drive to be useful" was redefined by these groups as both a drive to individual self-realization as well as a need to be with and for others. It was at once a reaching out to find the way one may exist within the nexus of a family or a community and a reaching in, the seeking of those associations and abilities that will make that person more. As members of these groups pointed out, neither of these tentative definitions excluded those with physical or cognitive deficits, the child with CP who communicates with the assistance of a computer or the person with Down syndrome whose strengths may be interpersonal.

All medicine can do is stabilize that patient, ending his or her immediate physical distress. That is not, however, a reason to discontinue care, group members agreed, even if that young CP patient's life is necessarily restricted and his or her life expectancy foreshortened. The qualities of humanness and personhood and the staff's resultant "duty to care" extend not simply to the physical patient, but more important to the person-in-relation, to a person who is the son or daughter of parents worried about a loved one. While each person in the discussion group valued those individual attributes that give most of us personality, drive, and a social posture, ultimately it was the fact of interpersonal association—between patient and patient family, on the one hand, and on the other between staff members and patient or patient family members—that was the most crucial aspect of a person's humanity. It was that which each, in the end, felt obliged to work toward in their care.

The citizens group members agreed wholeheartedly. In a powerful moment, the woman whose infant had died of anencephaly argued that interpersonal criteria were the essential component of humanness, and of the sanctity of human life doctrine's corollary, the duty to care. "To me, this whole thing boils down to two questions," she said. "How do we define what is human, and secondly, how does being human impact other human beings around us, and how do we fit into that social structure?" These were, she said, intimately related and not distinct questions. Whatever the relative strength of any individual criterion, the determination of commonality will impact upon others, both those who the person is associated with and within society at large.

The position returned by this examination is distinct from the one dominating current bioethics. It is, however, one argued by Oliver Sacks in *Awakenings*, a book about his treatment of postencephalitis patients. "It is human relations which carry the possibility of proper being-in-the-world. Feeling the fullness of another person, as a person, reality is given to us by the reality of people; reality is taken from us by the unreality of unpeople; our sense of reality, of trust, of security is critically dependent on a human relation."[30] The crucial determinant to these group members was not a clinically defined deficit or limit alone, but the degree to which the fragile patient would, someday or sometime, be able to act with and in relation to other people. When the fact or potential of that relationship becomes problematic in cases of extreme disability, the fact of love and concern on the part of a family member for a loved one was sufficient, hospital and lay group members insisted, to assure and define what one physician called the "human spark," the humanity that all seek to foster professionally and to serve individually through their care.

It is in the context of family, of the parent who says "treat my baby," that clinical decisions are made and humanness ultimately defined. This was made clear in a revealing moment in the hospital group when the group was discussing how to refer to anencephalic infants. "I'd call the baby 'he' or 'she' out of sensitivity towards the parents," said a very religious pediatrician completing a fellowship in neonatology. "If I'm going to come to the conclusions that I think I'd like to come to—that somehow I'd like to use that baby's organs for transplantation, thus terminating the baby's life—the only way I'd do that is by regarding the baby as not a full human being. And, really, technically, I think the baby is an 'it.' I wouldn't use the language, though, because I find it offensive."

While the infant itself is not, to this physician, fully human, it's humanity—and thus its right to care—is derived from the love and the need of the parents who present it for treatment. He may suggest palliative care or offer to parents the consideration of organ transplant to benefit others. But if the parents say, as did Baby K's mother, "Save my baby," he will treat the infant on the basis of their appeal and the human personhood it endows. There is, at least in this case, what for want of a better term might be called "human personhood by association," an inclusion within the protected circle on the basis of a love, relation, and commitment evidenced by another for the fragile, whatever his or her capacities or limits.

Believing health care dollars limited, members of neither group wished to see precious resources wasted, to see public monies squandered on useless procedures. In both groups, however, participants expressed concern that financial restraints in health care were pushing society toward reducing humanity to a cost-benefit eugenic equation. Ultimately, members of both groups insisted these are not simply clinical issues that can be defined on the basis of outcome assessments. They are more centrally social definitions whose central theme lies in the preservation and nurturing of even the most fragile relationship between persons. For their part, hospital group members do not wish to treat futility, to labor for a patient whose life expectancy is limited, who will never be able to grow, mature, and say, "thank you." Who does? Privately, each has his or her own idea about humanness, its definition, and its applicability to their work. For most, anencephaly represents a case of such obviously limiting severity that many would, like this physician, see them as less than persons, as organs to be harvested. And yet when a mother brings a child to the hospital with a condition that can be stabilized, to do less than assist that parent and child together would be to violate their sense of the human relation itself.

THE BABY K DECISION

From this perspective one can agree and disagree simultaneously with Judge Hilton's decision in the *Baby K* case. The infant is not an "it," an unperson unworthy of care. The baby is a living human being, albeit one whose fragilities are extraordinarily severe. What distinguishes the anencephalic is not a shortened life span or the simple fact of extreme deficit. As Judge Hilton noted, AIDS-infected persons may face a foreshortened future, and the lack of higher brain activity does not automatically rule out continued treatment of others, for example, patients in long-term comas. In the present tense, however, the anencephalic needing ventilation is no more or less worthy than any infant brought to the emergency room by parents seeking care.

That said, however, the anencephalic is not a person like all others. He or she forever lacks the capacity for interaction, for love returned. The idiosyncrasies by which we all are differentiated over time, one from the other, are things he or she will not learn. Nor will that child ever perceive the visual world, will never understand our speech and music. The infant will never walk or talk both because his or her life span will be too short to learn these skills and because anencephaly's neurologic deficits limit those capacities. To the extent that we value these attributes, the anencephalic's deficiencies might legitimately limit aggressive as opposed to stabilizing levels of care. We may tolerate one or more of these limiting conditions, at least for a time, in adults who have suffered grievous head trauma or neurological illnesses because of what their lives have meant and mean to us. For some, this is reason enough to treat a person aggressively into the indefinite future. But as an infant, the weight of historical association is withheld from the anencephalic's case.

Had the model included alternatives—levels of medical treatment ranging from "do nothing" through palliative care, stabilizing care, and aggressive care—their application would have strongly argued for stabilizing but not aggressively treating the anencephalic infant. To do less would be to deny the baby's humanity, to do more would ignore the real differences that exist between this infant and the adult we know. Infants like Baby K would therefore not be seen, by these participants, as candidates for the extraordinary medical measures with which both sentient adults and otherwise healthy infants are often treated. The anencephalic would not be a candidate for heart surgery, for example, or for organ transplantation. The infant's future is too truncated and its limits so manifest that such treatment would not serve the infant, his or her family, or society at large. But to do less than stabilize the infant's breathing and permit the infant's existence to continue through the provision of ventilator assistance would be to deny the humanity we purport to cherish and seek to preserve.

Like the findings of the organ transplant eligibility discussion groups, the results of these deliberations have been summarized, returned to participants for their comments, and are to be revised as a set of guidelines to be subjected to more traditional policy-making procedures. Even if the principles are broadly accepted, however, clear questions will remain. If emergency use of ventilation is "stabilizing," for example, will long-term ventilator use be similarly mandated? Will the continued withdrawal of funding for health care result in a shifting definition by future group participants, a "triage" mentality whose effect would be to draw the line between human and less-than-human more sharply for the purposes of cost accountancy?

"We are all contextualists," one physician said in his group. Each case is a complex balance of medical potential, patient need, family perspective, and hospital realities, he explained. Decisions must be made, case by case, balancing these and perhaps other factors. Citizen group members are less burdened with the fine distinctions between diagnoses and treatment alternatives. Their context is simultaneously personal, "How would I feel?" and social, "What should we do?" Ultimately, it may be that nonprofessionals will be involved in the first stage of this discursive process but that the application of clinical alternatives, guided by their judgment, will be reserved for professionals (bioethicists, nurses, physicians, pastoral counselors, etc.) with a background in the field.

This will neither violate the spirit of inclusion that this process advances nor the utility of the judgments returned. The latter offers broad social and communal guidelines for the decisions that must be made, in the end, by medical professionals with family members, and where possible, the patient him-or herself. As participants in the citizens group considering organ transplant eligibility and the criterion—compliance—made clear, however, there are limits to the nonprofessional's knowledge. Most have no direct experience with anencephaly, trisomy 18, or a host of other specific conditions. Nor are nonprofessionals more than dimly aware of the balancing act clinicians perform between potential treatment and the possible effect of those treatments. They do not wish to usurp the physician's role or the nurse's expertise. But to the extent that these are social as well as clinical concerns, they have insight and a wealth of other experiences that bear generally if not specifically on the context of medical decision making. And it is in this arena, one of boundaries and general definitions, that their views are at least equally insightful and of equal value to those of the clinician.

VALIDATION

This was a more difficult, less concrete exercise than its predecessor. In the context of absolute scarcity dominating organ transplant eligibility, the need for a choice between persons is clear. Here, however, the goal was defining criteria contributing to humanness, a philosophical construct with practical implications. Participants were caught between concrete examples—this anencephalic baby, that infant with CP—and a level of discourse that often was at once deeply personal and yet extremely difficult to articulate. One way to evaluate both the model and its utility is to see if it explains phenomena that otherwise have seemed inexplicable.

Lawrence J. Schneiderman and Sharyn Manning surveyed forty-three U.S. children's hospitals and asked if they were familiar with the *Baby K* case and if so what did they think of the decision.[31] More important, they then asked if each responding hospital would reject treatment for an anencephalic infant presenting with respiratory distress and if the *Baby K* case had affected hospital policy in such instances. The response was unanimous and unanimously equivocal. On the one hand, they reported, "Not one respondent endorses the life-sustaining treatment of Baby K." All their respondents called that judgment dumb, ridiculous, inappropriate, and outrageous. And yet, they collectively recalled twenty-eight patients whom they believed were similarly kept alive at their hospitals because of parental demands for treatment of the children. These were patients with severe brain damage, trisomy 13, trisomy 18, and a series of other conditions that were both limiting and likely to be fatal sooner rather than later. "In other words, although the physicians interviewed claimed that maintaining life support for an anencephalic baby was not acceptable practice, neither they nor the hospitals were inclined to establish non-treatment as customary practice, or test their expert opinion in the courts."[32]

The authors of that article did not attempt to explain this peculiar gulf between medical judgment and a pattern of ongoing clinical action at participants' hospitals that those same clinicians termed "outrageous" and "inappropriate." The deliberations of this group suggest a rationale, however. Simply, one may treat a person loved by others, a human person by association, even where clinical judgment suggests that clinical intervention will do no more than stabilize a fragile and failing life. "It is the function of medication, or surgery, or appropriate physiological procedures to rectify mechanism," Oliver Sacks observed, "the mechanism, the mechanisms, which are so deranged in these patients."[33] When a patient cannot be returned to normalcy, when no treatment will do more than stabilize a fragile and failing life, the function of medicine is limited and its practitioners will see the performance of their craft as futile.

Ventilating a patient like Baby K may stabilize the infant but cannot cure its condition. From the perspective of mechanism, the severely anencephalic infant is not a being like you or me. Similarly, the senior with advanced Alzheimer's disease, or the trauma patient in a permanent vegetative state is not the same person he or she was in days of health and ability. Nothing will rectify the mechanism of their bodies any more than stabilizing the severely disabled infant with CP—who has "aspirated one more time"—will result in long-term health or even long-term improvement. And so from a perspective of mechanistic medicine, treatment in all these cases is senseless.

But physicians are more than body mechanics, medicine is more than anatomy. Hospital professionals perceive and react to the pain of the relative who sees in the disabled infant or the comatose stroke-effected senior more than a problem to be defined through simple "outcome assessments." That patient with severe restrictions and a limited future becomes to them a human being by association through the many tasks of caring he or she requires. Their personhood is evidenced by those family members who love and care for them. Whatever a fragile patient's level of activity and performance—however limited his or her potential for physical improvement—that patient is a person, a human being whose status is affirmed by both the staff and the family members whose lives are defined in turn by that fragile being's continuance.

Often, a fragile patient's humanity, and thus the necessity for his or her care, is based upon the clinician's perception of the "human spark," which while flickering, is felt by the physician, nurse, or pastoral counselor who stands by that individual's bedside. "I have a shared meaning with this . . . entity," the pastoral counselor said in our group. "I can't remove myself." And so while medical personnel may suggest to the family that care will be only a brief reprieve, that futurity is an impossible goal, they will accept the humanity assigned by family members—or defined in the acts of daily medical care—and proceed in accord with that judgment.

Baby K Redux

Here is the answer to the riddle of Baby K, to the legal arguments over questions of treatment for those whose conditions impose severe physical and temporal limits on their existence. The anencephalic infant and the adult with active AIDS are different. With the latter we have history, while relationships with the former are both briefer and more elemental. The person with AIDS is a person we know, with whom we may empathize, and one whose ongoing relationship to others in our world is manifest. But as a rule of treatment in medical decision making we do not treat the historical person alone; the past weighed less strongly than the future in the groups' judgments. Nor are our decisions made only on the basis of a being's potential future service to itself or to others. Uncertain future is promise and potential, hope but not necessarily reality. Its im-

portance palls against the immediacy of the present. The focus of treatment decision making is and must be the son or daughter, the husband
or wife, the neighbor in extremes at the moment. To do less than care
denies them and those who love them, and perhaps, ourselves as well.

This is not what students are taught in medical or nursing schools or
what is urged by experts in bioethics debates over the nature of "futility."
Nor is it an "existential medicine" drawing its potency from what Oliver
Sacks called the "latent will, the agent, the 'I,' [with power], to call out
its commanding and coordinating powers."[34] That is the medicine of discrete individuality, of persons who are defined solely as autonomous, dis-
cretely physical beings. Its perspective fails, in the end, to the degree a
fragile patient, limited physically and in terms of a future, presents in a
clinic or the emergency room as a member of a family and of the community at large. And so while members of these or other discussion
groups, like Schneiderman and Mannings' survey respondents, may rail
against "futile" treatment of the limited person, the "it," they will continue to treat the person whose humanity is defined by the "we" of association, of familial care and affection within a societal context.

This may be a peculiarly Canadian perspective. Canada's national
health care program has long reflected a perspective based upon community support for the fragile, on social support for all those in need of
treatment and care. It also may be, however, that the valuation of communal over individual values, of present need over either future potential
or past performance reflects a more general social perspective that is not
merely Canadian but, instead, North American and perhaps international. I believe the latter to be true. The advantage of this approach is
that my suspicion can be tested using this hierarchy in other venues in a
way that is comparable and comprehensible.

7

Principled Limits: Medicine and Ethics

A congregation of disparate persons—health professionals, stakeholders, and representative citizens—met in a series of small-scale focus groups, reviewed a series of criteria defining elements of one or another real problem, and reached agreement on their relative importance. This is hopeful and itself worthy of note. It is no small achievement to find substantial unanimity across the supposedly conflicting views and values of a "hospital culture's" diverse congregation of physicians, nurses, ethicists, pastoral counselors, and social workers. That their general conclusions were shared in the main by stakeholders and by other citizens is almost unprecedented.

What was truly remarkable, however, was that across these groups positions were discussed and judgments made without anyone ever standing on principle, asserting their own or another's rights, or taking recourse behind a catch-all phrase like "futility," "outcome assessment," or even "quality of life." The paradoxical flavor of traditional debates that revolve around the definition of principled nouns or noun phrases like "futility," "life," "humanness," "personhood," and so forth, was also largely absent from these deliberations. In large part this results from the multicriterion perspective permitting the consideration of a range of priorities rather than an either/or formulation. Further, in traditional, principle-based bioethics, "every moral agent is, at base, symmetrically positioned with respect to every morally considerable being—everyone's needs and interests have precisely the same pull on everyone else."[1] In the complexities of medical decision making, things are rarely equal, however. By permitting overlapping valuations in the evaluation of multiple criteria, which may all impact in varying degrees upon a specific goal, a more realistic portrait of the importance of both clinical criteria and social values was returned.

What resulted was not consensus, if by that what is meant is a seamless, collective opinion. Differences remained within groups whose members disagreed on some priorities and on some issues. In both programs, individual groups reached slightly different valuations, albeit usually in discussion of level-2 and especially level-3 criteria. These occurred because, at times, different focus groups operated from different definitions, and thus in their deliberations meant different things in discussing supposedly clear criteria like "compliance." In the final analysis, this was significant and useful, a fact to be incorporated into rather than a barrier to a final consensual statement. There was general agreement on the broad parameters of the issues discussed. Where differences existed in defining criteria—differences that were previously unidentified in the literature—understanding those differences often uncovered areas of agreement rather than a bedrock of differing opinion. Here the discussion of "compliance" is an excellent example.

The moral intuitions of participants, the set of reflexive values each held and presented in the discussion, were often raised in one or another discussion. This doctor says an anencephalic is not human to him. It lacks the "spark" by which he defines humankind. Another whose brother has Down syndrome disagrees, as does a nurse worried that if anencephalics are excluded the fragile elderly will be too. "And so you'd kill Granny?" she asks. Down syndrome association participants say, in effect, "The fact of limits does not diminish the love our children, brothers, and sisters share, or their human worth." And yet, as members of a group and of society at large, participants balanced their personal beliefs and goals against other socially shared realities. In the crucible of these discussions, individual value systems were revealed and critiqued within the context of the problem at hand.

This is not to say the deliberations were not principled. Rather, the focus of the discussion was not on abstract principle but on the "assumptions and arguments"[2] that are the heart of a practical bioethics concerned with the concrete moral problems of care and care-based decisions in a community and society. The use of defining criteria in a prepared hierarchy helped assure discussion would be focused at a level where judgments were themselves tied to a more practical perspective. Like us all, group participants were concerned with fairness, with justice, and more

Figure 7.1
Faces in a Bowl

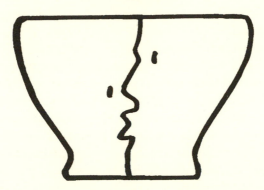

generally the consistent application of rules and moral assumptions they believed should determine the treatment of the fragile in society. Had the hierarchy included these values as criteria, they would certainly have been strongly endorsed. The sometimes intense deliberations focused, however, on means rather than ends, on the applicability of concrete criteria in a context where those values were background to rather than central figures of concern. In this process, both midlevel principles and the schemes of their application did play a part. Indeed, they were defined and reshaped by the dialogue that occurred within the crucible of these group discussions. But here they were revealed as personal values whose application is difficult and perhaps problematic in a clinical setting. "It is one thing to have values," said a psychiatrist in one focus group. "It's another to have to state and then apply them."

Rather than the featureless silhouettes of the visual illusion presented in chapter 3, (Figure 3.1), the result is one of recognizable faces joined within a general shape and context whose boundaries are clear (see Figure 7.1). No claimant must disappear for another to be perceived. The participants are not erased by attention to the body of principle that traditionally stands above and beyond the individual human person. In this analogy, principles and values become the lines of the goblet itself, the context in which the persons are perceived and their needs defined. This results from the redefinition of criteria in a more concrete manner, permitting both a clearer evaluation of claimants and the criteria that distinguish them within a social context.

This balances a traditional principled approach whose abstraction largely denies the lived reality of patients and medical personnel, neces-

sarily ignoring relations that exist between all parties in a medical dilemma. "The methods through which we most commonly advance and
assess ethical claims," says James Lindemann Nelson, "are clumsy at il-
luminating what's morally important about intimacy."[3] The realities of
interpersonal attachment, and of shared experiences and values, do not
coexist comfortably with principle's necessarily abstract generalizations.
And yet, decisions for or against care must be made by the parents,
spouses, and children of the fragile, by intimates whose interest and concern are the impetus of court challenges to hospital policy. For every
Helen Wanglie or Baby K is a spouse or parent who seeks to maintain a
person whose relation to the caregiver or surrogate is personally critical.
In the principled drive for impartiality, for abstract equality, and faceless
justice, the singular perceptions of a caregiver, patient, or patient surrogate are often viewed with suspicion, and thus discounted by those whose
views are based on a traditional philosophic approach.

The most significant findings returned by this work was the groups'
emphasis on the fragile, restricted patient as a person defined not by deficit
alone but also by his or her relationships with others and with society at
large. Treatment decisions are therefore to be directed not at the individual body alone but at the symptoms experienced by a person brought
to the hospital by a relative whose love and observations also define the
patient's personhood and resultant care. "Why do we keep on doing what
we're doing? It's the subjectivity of this interaction," a neonatologist said
of the parent bringing in a child with severe cerebral palsy who had
aspirated "one more time." As important, the fact of relation is limited
not to the patient's surrogate, but includes as well the medical professional
whose personal associations and values are invested in that patient's care.
"I have a shared meaning with this . . . entity," a pastoral counselor said.
"I can't remove myself."

What results is a definition of human personhood based not solely on
the characteristics of the discrete individual, and certainly not on clinically assessable criteria alone, but also on the thick, richly evident social
realities shared by fragile claimant and the healthy person alike. It is not
IQ test scores, an urgent condition ranking, or probability of survival
alone that should therefore define a person's eligibility as a transplant
candidate. These are signs signifying attributes that represent qualities
valued by society as a whole. Any criteria may or may not appropriately
represent the signified value. A large part of the AHP approach used in
earlier chapters had as its result the quantifiable statement of those values

and the inappropriateness of the signifiers now used to represent them. As Canadians argued popularly through the press, the limits imposed upon Terry Urquart by his Down syndrome were less important than his demonstrable abilities and the determination of the family and friends who stood willing and able to support him in his transplant candidacy. The care of Baby K was to be determined not by her extreme deficits alone, but also by her mother's insistence that her child's life was real, important, and worth fighting for. These are criteria not measured by current clinical or bioethical standards, and it is the distance between their importance—and the limits of those standard clinical tests—that often gives rise to public debate and court battle.

The principles of individuality and of individual autonomy are simply too narrow to encompass either the realities of modern medicine or the complex realities by which we live together and judge each other. As a result, issues of individual self-determination—the patient's right of "choice"—become a complex mediation between social, professional, personal, and familial concerns. This was made clear in the hospital groups' discussions of physical attributes. Participants were shocked when they learned from one discussant that some genetic counseling clients at the hospital were choosing to abort their fetuses when amniocentesis revealed their child would be born with a correctable cleft palate. Nobody doubted the mothers' "right" to make this determination under current law. But such an act violated, for most, a fundamental belief that physical appearance should not be the criteria by which we reject or accept a person into our circle.

Immanuel Kant's "respect for persons," which has become virtually synonymous with the principle of self-determination and autonomy, is redefined in this view as a *right-in-association*, one bounded not by individual prejudice or concern but by the greater relation of the decision maker to his or her community, to the object of those decisions within society at large. It is not, therefore, necessarily a matter of a right to do what one wants, but equally important the responsibility of choosing for another.

Thus the "right" of a person to abort a fetus because of a repairable cleft palate denies both responsibility to that potential person and to communal values defining appearance as the least of attributes that make a human being. Similarly, the parents of Baby Ross and Baby Doe had the right to deny surgery for a repairable abdominal atresia because those infants had Down syndrome. But permitting their death because the care of a child with differences is difficult to deny, their critics said, an associative value asserting humanness as a social rather than purely cognitive characteristic.

What results is a new definition of humanness and personhood that, in Mildred Z. Solomon's words, is "Understood as an essentially social self that is in constant relationship with others and with one's surroundings; not a static, highly rational ego determining its own private destiny, but a dynamic self shaped by and affecting others."[4] Whenever one makes choices for oneself or for others, the context of that decision is always first interpersonal and then social. Rights and obligations alike are based upon a circle of contingent relations defining a person's place within the social, medical, and professional circles.

It was this socially complex perspective that explained the differences of definition in assessing "compliance" as a criterion in organ transplant eligibility. For the first hospital group, the unary assumption of patient adherence to medical orders denied the complex process of staff, patient, and patient-family interaction that can advance or impede the act of compliance. It thus became, for professional participants, a measure of their ability to explain processes and procedural requests, as well as to understand that person's needs and contexts (familial, social, economic). For members of the Down Syndrome Family Association, however, compliance was perceived as measuring a person's willingness to participate wholly in a medical process whose scarce resources demand that each claimant do what he or she can to assure "the best bang for the buck," the best use of a transplantable human organ. Each from its own perspective, all groups saw compliance as measuring a process of negotiation and education between patient, family, and medical staff.

Similarly, IQ was devalued as a criterion in organ transplant eligibility, group participants said, because it does not measure what they perceived as important in a person. "I would think that involvement with others, ability to participate in society and to have a meaningful life would be more important," said a physician who acknowledged its current use at her hospital. "I know some very bright people who don't contribute very much, who have a very difficult time," said a member of the citizen group. The ability to participate in a shared society at one or another level is what participants wished to facilitate in the context of absolute scarcity. IQ as an indicator of a type of abstract intelligence simply did not reflect the broader range of cognitive attributes all wished to preserve and foster.

While all would insist on recognition for society's valuable members, for those whose life and work places them at the center of our shared worlds, none were sure how to define or quantify this. What all did know, however, was that "public recognition" was not the way they wanted this to be measured. The well-known actor, the superior athlete, the writer of best-selling novels may have contributed to our world, but that fact should not result in his or her automatic advancement on the organ transplant lists or in the hierarchy of humanness considered in chapter 6. Those things speak to the performance of the person, but not to his or her social life or personal relationships. And it is to those criteria that these participants were most committed.

Here the use of temporality, of past, present, and future tenses in level-1 criteria was critical. Some have suggested that health care must be based upon the person's potential contribution to society at large. Others believe what is most important is not present service but past performance. But across these groups the real issue, they said, was first and foremost the present condition of the patient who presents in distress. In the case of the anencephalic—or the CP patient who "aspirates one more time"— stabilizing treatment eliminates the problem without curing its underlying origin. But that outcome is sufficient when a parent asks for assistance for his or her child. The parent or caregiver's love and need is primary evidence of the interpersonal relation all seek to foster and thus of the humanity all ultimately are pledged to serve.

In the arena of organ transplant eligibility criteria, on the other hand, the problem is one of both the patient's future and that of the survival of the graft organ itself. Here, for most participants, longer is better. But because it is virtually impossible to predict long-term outcome, the importance of time differences flattens between five and ten years. And for those with little likelihood of surviving more than a year or two even with a new organ, the exercise would be almost wasteful of that organ.

An essential perspective of these judgments is that the resource that medicine and society must seek to preserve is neither a scarce resource to be maximized nor the discrete, autonomous individual it is presumed to serve. Where a resource is not and cannot be made sufficient for all, there is a respect for the resource itself—for example, the graft organ. Its importance, however, is derived from its potential to preserve the person-in-association. The participants in these groups thus argue that the primary, principled resource of society does not reside in the family and community member whose continuance sustains us communally. Criteria defining an ethical program of allocation must serve this general definition first. This perspective stands in strong juxtaposition to the individually based, typically utilitarian approach of many contemporary ethicists and bioethicists.

What is returned to in these judgments is an older view of medicine. It is not simply an objective clinical exercise in which tests both define problems and result in decisions based on objective standards. It is more complex than that. As perceived by professional and lay members of these focus groups, medicine is a deeply social, interpersonal effort involving a rich series of connections and associations: staff-patient, patient-family, family-doctor, doctor-staff, staff-patients, family, all written against the background of a society that enables or inhibits care and caring in their broadest sense. Its goal is not the exclusive address of a disease's presence and symptoms, but the health of the patient in the context of family and community. This changes the context of technical medicine in many circumstances, especially those involving extreme illness and the outer limits of modernity's evolving technological expertise.

This conclusion in and of itself has clinical ramifications. Several years ago I counseled informally an emergency room nurse who railed against the persons who she helped treat, day by day. So much of the ER's work was wasted and useless, she said. I'm tired, she told me, of struggling to stabilize the old who having suffered a serious heart attack or stroke, of getting someone who is deathly ill through one more crisis. Where's the benefit, she asked. What's it all for? The street person with pneumonia will be back in a month with another debilitating and probably life-threatening condition. The heart attack patient will infarct again. And of course the survivor of a serious stroke almost surely will suffer another and next time bleed fatally. Why save someone to a diminished and sometimes *severely* diminished state? It's useless, she told me. Non-sensical.

If the purpose of medicine was solely curative, she was clearly correct. If its orientation is only future based, her ER was indeed a wasteful place. I argued, however, that she does not see what the extra days or weeks won for excessively fragile patients mean to them and their families. The week of our discussions I had been with a woman when her stepfather suffered a massive heart attack. Although the damage was extreme, an ER team had worked long and hard to stabilize him. In the days immediately following his heart attack, he had time to meet with his family and to plan with them for their future; to say goodbye. Five days after his initial admission he died, but those five days were critical to them all. The labors of the ER team members who treated this man were not wasted. The time won by their efforts was enormously important to this patient and to his family. But it was this result, the use made of the present time extended, that the ER nurse never saw. The old sneer, "The operation was a success, but the patient died," was reversed in this event. "The patient died, but the operation was a success," because it served patient and family members in significant ways.

PRINCIPLED ARGUMENT

Program participants utilized a complex system of evaluation in addressing the goals of these two hierarchies. Within the MCDM context, they cobbled together an approach combining elements of a variety of philosophic traditions typically assumed to be distinct. These included casuistry,[5] arguing from individual case; contextualism, sometimes called the "new pragmatism;"[6] an implicit constructivism, developing a meaning that has clinical and moral implications;[7] outcome assessment, seeking the maximal use of scarce resources; and discourse ethics' *modus operandi*, sustained discussion in an attempt to find an answer to a specific problem.[8]

The whole project was flavored by the new pragmatism, whose advocates argue, "The rejection of deduction from grand and universal principles in favor of detailed attention to context, empirical realities, and differences among individuals and groups."[9] But so, too, was the discussion itself. Participants were focused upon the consideration of issues within the context of budgetary constraints, political realities, social principles, and the real differences that exist within the complexities of modern medical situations. Members of every group argued from cases they knew, either from hospital rounds and shared consultation or from personal experience. In defining the importance of IQ, for example, the positive experience of participants with persons of Down syndrome, and with persons whose high IQ scores resulted neither in a likable personality nor in a social contribution they admired, weighed heavily in the discussion. All availed themselves of the shared context of the news. Members discussing organ transplantation reviewed a range of cases— Mickey Mantle to Sandra Jensen—for their bearing on the problem of determining eligibility. In their discussions of humanness, they discussed everything from anencephaly to the coma of a citizen participant's father-in-law.

This does not mean they argued individual cases while ignoring the structural factors that make one or another case representative of more general concerns and social issues. Participants in every group were alive to the social, political, and organizational elements affecting the issues they sought to address. If a family has no recourse to expert home care, then a person with extreme disabilities will be at longer-term risk if he or she is returned home after surviving a medical crisis. Should the Canadian commitment to free medical care be retracted, then issues of individual financial resources would be more important than they are today to these participants. Finally, members of all groups were concerned with outcome, with seeking the best possible result for the patient within the context of increasingly scarce resources.

All this occurred within the framework of a type of discourse ethics, one whose basic assumption is that only together can persons reach an understanding about a problem or an issue. But while discourse ethics seeks an approximation of truth, the goal here was more modest. What was returned by these discussions was a portrait of what participants believed correct within the context of their knowledge and the realities of both the medical system they know and the social system that supports it: this is, for want of a better term, a regional ethics whose proximate truths are built on an understanding of assumptions and arguments—both practical and principled—but limited to and only operative at the level of the community.

There is no guarantee, for example, that the conclusions of the Toronto focus groups will be those a Vancouver, B.C. or Halifax, N.S. community would accept. Given the differences between U.S. and Canadian medical systems, and their differing views of communal versus individual values, it is likely that at least some of the criteria in both models would be ranked differently by hospital and community groups in, for example, Dallas, Texas, or Beloxi, Mississippi. And yet, this only says that we interpret data differently based upon the cultural ethos and social prejudices of our disparate communities. Medical ethics is not independent of local and regional values and restraints. In application, universal principles are as much cultural artifacts as they are philosophic abstract truths.

Even if discussion groups at all hospitals in all cities where transplants are performed agreed that patient (and graft) survival was the crucial, first criterion for all organs, that conclusion would still be proximate, not universal—and certainly not eternal. Instead, it would be a conclusion bounded by the context of the debate and the age in which it was carried out. Because one says, today, "we believe this" does not mean that in a hundred years—or even in twenty—that value or principle will remain in favor. The long history briefly detailed in chapter 2 was thus the history of bounded, regionally based truths accepted and rejected, time and again, as our Western culture grew and matured.

What resulted from this exercise was a practical ethics grounded in the concrete but moving toward the general level of social policy. Participants began not with an overriding principle to be applied reflexively but with a sense of reciprocity and relation ultimately defining, for them, the place of the fragile in the community we all share. From this they extrapolated, using personal experience and the social preference of highly publicized cases, to move toward a general position that may contribute to practical care guidelines. This type of approach was perhaps most akin to Michael Walzer's view of an ethical or moral vision that is "thick from the beginning, culturally integrated, fully resonant,"[10] one that takes on the language of abstract principle and formal right or obligation only when it needs a justification.

This inversion of the traditional progression from thin to thick—from the principled to the practical—was facilitated, encouraged, and perhaps necessitated by the AHP and the hierarchies created for participant review. That does not mitigate the power of the approach or the degree to which it permitted a range of persons to discuss shared problems and then reach a level of substantial agreement. Think of it as the anthropology that Kant once argued is a necessary component of any metaphysics of morals. In the section entitled the Doctrine of Virtue he argued in *Metaphysics of Morals* that insofar as we are rational beings, those attempting to work out issues of human morality require an investigative, anthropologic "science of man."[11] The potential of an anthropology of ethics, largely ignored by principle-based ethicists (and, practically, by Kant himself), is enabled by the MCDM approach advocated here. The result has been a series of judgments contributing to the definition of socially bounded, operational principles and to an implicit critique of their use as explanatory totems within a specific clinical context.

From this exercise things were learned. The goal of consensus is not foredoomed, for example, if by consensus we mean agreement on the relation between criteria defining a problem set. That accord will reflect not just abstract principle or purportedly universal truths, however, but a general perspective of a clearly defined group or culture. The greater goal of medical philosophy, "A comprehensive and coherent moral theory for medical practice based on universal principles applying to all and capable of justifying particular lines of conduct in individual cases," remains unfulfilled.[12] Indeed, it is likely that goal can never be realized because it assumes the existence of universal and universally applicable

principles. Our views and values are simply too different, and the economic and social contexts that contribute to and are simultaneously in-
fluenced by them are too important a part of the broad equation of ethical
analysis and response.

To the degree that agreement is possible, the potential for bioethics to
serve as a communal rather than a professional resource is announced.
Since its birth as a subset of medical philosophy, bioethics has explored
"the moral obligations of health professionals and society in meeting the
needs of the sick and injured."[13] Official bioethics was created by and for
professionals whose deliberations are then supposedly passed to a patient
who is to be guided by its principled stance. As Donald C. Ainslie acutely
observed, however, "Issues concerning professional ethics and the role of
the state in funding and regulating the health professions define the
boundaries of bioethics. But . . . since questions of professional ethics are
not always insulated from the questions those living with disease confront
in their everyday lives, it is sometimes impossible to answer the former
questions without taking a stand on the latter ones."[14] That is to say the
principles that may guide professional behavior do not necessarily answer
the needs, concerns, or perceptions of the patient or caregiver him- or
herself. Reversing the order of knowing by allowing from the start the
input of a variety of stakeholders offers the potential for a more inclusive,
more realistic medical ethics.

An unexpected boon of this approach was its potential as an educational tool. Members of all groups found the experience of hierarchical
evaluation humbling and enlightening. One physician came to the first
group with a list of professional journal articles he had pulled from the
hospital's library. "I'll play this game," he said, "but if someone wants to
know the answers I've got the papers here." But the arguments in those
journal articles did not answer the practical concerns of other group participants. Nor did they speak to the social issues he and his colleagues
had to address in the discussion group and each working day. For him
and for others, the discussion group exercise forced a bridge joining social
issues and preconceived values, approaches of the general literature, the
need to defend and argue a position in terms of specific concrete criteria
and cases.

Members of the citizen groups were educated in other ways. Making
decisions in the context of medical uncertainty was for some a disturbing
experience. In the Down Syndrome Association meeting, for example,
one person said, "This is hard. I don't want to make these judgments!"
Another person reminded her that judgments are being made, day by day,

in hospitals and elsewhere. "That's what this is about," she said. "It's what doctors and others are doing." Participation in the nonprofessional focus groups gave lay group members an idea of the real and complex dilemmas faced by doctors, nurses, and other medical decision makers. The lesson that sometimes decisions must be, and that those who make them must agonize over the choices they present, was new information for many nonhospital participants. And, of course, like the participating health professionals, they were required to examine their own reflexive assumptions within the context of social needs and obligations.

OTHER APPROACHES

Others have used various techniques to seek new answers to problematic medical issues in recent years. Since one aim of this work has been methodological, identifying better ways to address bioethical dilemmas, it is useful to note in passing the relation of other attempts to the MCDM approach advanced here. Two deserve special consideration, the first for its real impact and the second for its academic interest. The well-discussed Oregon experiment in medical rationing, for example, used a public committee to prioritize a long list of medical procedures paid for with public monies.[15] Basic care was given preference over expensive procedures— bone marrow transplantation, for example—whose outcome was often uncertain. Among those who thus were denied potentially life-saving treatment was an attractive, seven-year-old boy, Coby Howard, for whom bone marrow transplant was denied.[16] Was this the best way to handle a finite budget, people asked? Must a young boy be allowed to die even when salvation is potentially available?[17] Is medicine really just a matter of cost-benefit analysis, and are the advantages of advanced modern technology only for those wealthy enough to afford private medical insurance or to directly pay for one or another procedure?

Because in theory all Canadians have equal access to all medical procedures, the Oregon program would be unacceptable in this country. Even in the United States, some believed its apparent two-tier standard based on economic means—those with private insurance or means could pay for treatment denied patients relying on public health insurance—violated principles of equitable access and just treatment for all. Certainly its approach denies the exigent case, the unusual circumstance, and perhaps most important, the relation between person and interpersonal community. How can one balance lives that may be saved by immunization with lives of those who face life-threatening conditions today, persons of the community for whom expensive but potentially effective treatments are available?

One can question the Oregon experiment's approach on the basis of its goal, maximizing limited health dollars. As Robert M. Veatch points out, "an unexpectedly strong case can be made for 'big ticket' [expensive] items both as innovative trial therapies and as research to benefit future generations, especially when the focus is on persons who are or will be among the worst off."[18] But the real problem may be the goal itself. Is the limited time frame of a budget year the one that should be used in life and death decision making? If the goal is not economic—maximizing health care dollars—but medical "care for the fragile," other possibilities may present themselves. Sometimes the hardest part of modeling such problems is in defining the goal, in choosing one that does not imbed the perspective and resultant criteria that will deny needed structural change.

More recently, several British physicians in general practice concerned about the difficulty of doing their best for each individual patient in a context of shrinking health resources, developed a policy defining how they would ration health care services to their patients. "If the partnership has to choose which of two patients should have priority in receiving some beneficial and expensive treatment," they reported, it would endorse "fair innings"— discriminating against seniors—and consider patient responsibility for his or her illness as criteria affecting clinical recommendations.[19] But, they announced, the medical partners also would reject both "the value of a patient to society" and "the value of a patient's life to that patient" as applicable criteria.[20]

Why one criterion and not another? "If they had to choose between a saint and a rotter," one commentator asked, "each of equal age and without dependents, then how would they solve the crisis?"[21] As important, perhaps, what would these practitioners say to the patient who, denied treatment on the basis of their policy, learned that doctors down the road offered a different set of priorities? "You mean, because you're my doctor I don't get this treatment while another doctor might make a different judgment? Send me there!"

With other commentators, Loyola University bioethicist Dave Thomasma, praised both the physicians' attempt to rationally consider alternatives in a context of scarcity and then to present them to the public. Thomasma also noted approvingly that "morally, good rationing occurs when allocation is based on public criteria."[22] This assumes, first that "rationing" on the basis of economic criteria is ever good, and second, that one can know what those public criteria might be. In this case, the physicians made their judgments without public input or discussion. They met with a bioethicist to discuss the principles that would guide the policies they wished to formulate. Patients were not consulted.

British physicians may serve as "philosopher kings," unilaterally making exclusionary decisions on the basis of personal perspectives. In litigious North America, however, the atypical judgments of individual physicians and hospitals boards are almost routinely referred to the courts for review. Regal professional judgment does not rule in the United States or in Canada. This is almost certainly for the best because few physicians on either side of the Atlantic are trained for an imperial role. As Dr. Arthur Caplan, director of the Center for Bioethics as the University of Pennsylvania stated flatly: "They're not equipped to make [such] judgments."[23] The approach advocated here opens the discussion of patient care to those who will be most affected by resulting policy. Patients can be invited to participate in the process, either using a hierarchy created by (or outside facilitators), physicians, or in the creation of the hierarchy itself. In this way a program that is inclusive rather than exclusive can be enjoined from the start.

Like the Oregon experiment, the Asbury draft policy assumes the reality of scarcity and the resulting necessity of limiting treatment on the basis of abstractions whose human reality is carefully obscured. Who is to say what age is too old? How is "responsibility" to be defined? Will the forty-five or fifty-year-old father be denied treatment so his four-year-old son can receive it? If each physician sets practice policies based on his or her own principled set, where is the equity most insist must exist across a system?

At a different level, the assumption of limited resources—which was the impetus for both programs—is itself an assumption whose tenets are flexible. One of the lessons learned in the debate over hemodialysis in the 1960s was that such economic limits are relative, not absolute. Governments can decide to fund expensive procedures for all, to assure equality across the health care system at either a basic or an advanced level. Scarcity in this context is not a given but the result of public decisions that themselves represent values and choices. And so the assumptions of these models express values and principles that, in the end, may limit the goals of the medical ethicists themselves.

CONCLUSION

It is necessary to end upon a note of incompleteness, of promises unfulfilled and problems unresolved. An MCDM approach is not a magic
wand that will instantly resolve all issues facing medical ethics today. The
importance of both the Oregon experiment and the Asbury policy statement resides in the dangers inherent in modeling, in the choice of well-
articulated goals and clearly related criteria when defining a problem and
then searching for its solution. Indeed, one of the advantages of the approach presented here is the exercise of modeling itself, of defining a
specific goal and its contributing criteria.

In constructing a hierarchy of criteria contributing to a clearly stated
goal, one necessarily incorporates social and cultural perspectives whose
values remain embedded in it. Because our morality and ethics begin with
thickly textured experience and social values and then extends to the
level of theory, the Analytic Hierarchy Process and other MCDM approaches clarify the values and prejudices we bring to a problem. They
will not necessarily transform moral debate into societal consensus. Nor
do they guarantee optimal solutions. In the end, these are simply methodologies useful to the degree they provide a way of expressing the com-
ponents of the moral and ethical intuition we apply as people and as a
community. In some contexts, these approaches may be sufficient to define a problem and evaluate its criteria in a way that will lead to agreement
among the many participants in a problem or issue. In others, it likely
will not.

What is clear, I believe, is that the perspective of traditional philosophy
will not serve in the coming decades. Indeed, it does not serve us well
today. Abstract principle has never been easily applied to concrete issues,
and as societies grew in complexity and technological power, their applicability diminished accordingly. At the least, what the MCDM approach advanced here offers is a bridge between principle and practice,
between policy without reference to person and the narrow perspective
of an individual's case. At best, it offers the potential for a medical ethics
whose focus is on both the goal of medicine and the realities of medical
practice within a community and a society.

This is not, however, a cause for despair. The potential exists for a
bioethics that stands between today's opposing views of, on the one hand,
libertarian individualism, and on the other, radical communitarianism.
The first insists all issues must be decided on the basis of individual rights

and the second on the insistence of a common shared vision. Both are right. Neither wholly serves. The individual exists in a community, is shaped by a series of interpersonal associations, and is treated (or abandoned) by the society in which he or she lives. Communities do not suffer illnesses, people do. To adequately address the bioethical issues facing us—as patients, professionals, and as a community-at-large—what is needed is an approach that will be grounded in the concrete, both the reality of the patient and that of the community ultimately responsible for his or her care or noncare. What is proposed here is a methodology that permits both levels to be perceived simultaneously and perhaps inclusively. To the extent that potential is enabled, and the links between "thick" and "thin" moral actions are revealed, paradoxical problems can be first restated and then reinterpreted in a way that makes them no less difficult but at the least more manageable. The potential for their resolution thus becomes possible.

Notes

CHAPTER 1

1. Shana Alexander, They decide who lives, who dies, *Life Magazine*, November 9, 1962.

2. Nancy S. Jecker, Caring for "socially undesirable" patients, *Cambridge Quarterly of Healthcare Ethics* (1996): 5:4, 500–510.

3. A. H. Proctor Katz, Social-psychological characteristics of patients receiving hemodialysis treatment for chronic renal failure. Public Health Service, Kidney Disease Control Program, July 1969, quoted in Jecker, caring for "socially undesirable" patients.

4. *Congressional Record*, September 30, 1972, 33,004–33,008.

5. Philip R. Reilly, *The Surgical Solution: A History of Involuntary Sterilization in the United States* (Baltimore: Johns Hopkins University Press, 1991).

6. Martin S. Pernick, *The Black Stork: Eugenics and the Death of "Defective" Babies in American Medicine and Motion Pictures Since 1915* (New York: Oxford University Press, 1995).

7. D. Sudnow, *Passing On* (Englewood Cliffs, N.J.: Prentice Hall, 1967), 101. Also quoted in Jecker, Caring for "socially undesirable" patients.

8. Robert M. Veatch, Should basic care get priority? Doubts about rationing the Oregon way, *Kennedy Institute of Ethics Journal* (1991): 1:3, 187–206; Harvey D. Klevit et al., Prioritization of health care services: A progress report by the Oregon Health Services commission, *Archives of Internal Medicine* (1991): 151; 912–16.

9. Albert R. Jonsen. The birth of bioethics, *Hastings Center Report*, Special Supplement (November-December 1993), S1.

10. Susan M. Wolf, Shifting paradigms in bioethics and health law: The rise of a new pragmatism, *American Journal of Law and Medicine* (1994): 20:4, 395–415.

11. Howard Brody, Assisted death—a compassionate response to medical failure, *New England Journal of Medicine* (1992): 327, 124–28, quoted in David Thomasma, An analysis for and against euthanasia and assisted suicide, Part 1. *Cambridge Quarterly of Healthcare Ethics* (1996): 5:1, 62–76.

12. Wolf, Shifting paradigms in bioethics and health law, 403.

13. John Lantos, Seeking justice for Priscilla, *Cambridge Quarterly of Healthcare Ethics* (1996): 5:4, 489.

14. John Horgan, Eugenics revisited, *Scientific American*, (June 1993): 122–31.

15. Peter Singer, *Rethinking Life and death: The Collapse of Our Traditional Ethics* (New York: St. Martin's Press, 1995), 188. Whether this doctrine was ever a consistent guide is another issue entirely. See T. Koch, Does the sanctity of human life doctrine sanctify humanness, or life? *Cambridge Quarterly of Healthcare Ethics*, in press.

16. After winning the 1994 Nobel Prize, Kenzaburo Oe said he was quitting fiction because he had completed his mission: to speak somehow for his severely brain-damaged son, Hikari. For a review of Oe's work, mission, and his views of the "birth defective," see D. Remnick, Reading Japan, *New Yorker*, February 6, 1995, 38–43.

17. Oliver Sacks' work on the capabilities of the neurologically damaged is central to these questions. See, for example, Oliver Sacks, *The Man Who Mistook His Wife for a Hat* (New York: Summit Books, 1985), section four; Oliver Sacks, *An Anthropologist on Mars* (New York: Knopf, 1995), 188–204.

18. Horgan, Eugenics revisited, 122–31.

19. Daniel Callahan, *Setting Limits: Medical Goals in an Aging Society* (New York: Simon and Schuster, 1987).

20. Laurence H. Tribe, *Abortion: The Clash of Absolutes* (New York: W. W. Norton & Co., 1990).

21. Margaret A. Somerville, Reproductive technologies, euthanasia, and the search for a new societal paradigm, *Social Science and Medicine* (1996): 42:12, ix–xii.

22. Wolf, Shifting paradigms in bioethics and health law, 395–415.

23. Albert R. Jonsen, Casuistry: An alternative or complement to principles? *Kennedy Institute of Ethics Journal* (1995): 5:3, 237–51.

24. Henk A. Ten Have, Medical technology assessment and ethics—Ambivalent relations, *Hastings Center Report* (1995): 25:5, 13–19.

25. Jonsen, Casuistry: An alternative or compliment to principles, 237.

26. For a review of the impact of these cases, see John Lantos, Baby Doe five years later: Implications for child health, *New England Journal of Medicine* (1987): 317, 444–47; G. Y. York, R. M. Ballarno, and R. O. York, Baby Doe regulations and medical judgment, *Social Science and Medicine* (1990): 30, 657–64.

27. Evert Van Leeuwen and Gerrit K. Kimsma, Acting or letting go: Medical decision making in neonatology in the Netherlands, *Cambridge Quarterly of Heathcare Ethics* (1993): 2, 265–69.

28. *In re Conservatorship of Wanglie*, No. PX-91–283 (Minn. Dist. Ct. Prob. Div. July 1, 1991).

29. *Roe v. Wade*, 410 US 113 (1973).

30. Peter Gould, The tyranny of taxonomy, *The Sciences* (May/June 1982): 7–9.

31. David Hume, *An Inquiry Concerning the Principles of Morals* (1777), quoted in Amy Gutmann and Dennis Thompson, *Democracy and Disagreement* (Cambridge, Mass.: Harvard University Press, 1996), 21. David Hume assumed that conditions of extreme scarcity do not result in moral conflicts, a position that would seem to be challenged by issues arising from organ transplant eligibility discussed in chapters 4 and 5.

32. Stephen G. Post, *The Moral Challenge of Alzheimer Disease* (Baltimore: Johns Hopkins University Press, 1995).

33. Abel A. Fernandez, Expert choice: Software review, *OR/MS Today* (Online Edition) (1996): 23:4.

34. Arthur L. Caplan, What bioethics brought to the public, *Hastings Center Report*, Special Supplement (November/December 1993): S14.

35. Tom Koch, Normative and prescriptive criteria: The efficacy of organ transplantation allocation protocols. *Theoretical Medicine* (1996): 17:1, 77–78.

36. M. Benjamin, C. Cohen, and E. Grochowski, What transplantation can teach us about health care reform, *New England Journal of Medicine* (1994): 330: 12, 858–60.

37. See, for example, David A. Stupf, The infant with anencephaly, *New England Journal of Medicine* (1990): 322, 669.

38. See, for example, *In re T.A.C.P.* 609 So. 2d 588, 589 (Florida, 1992). This aspect of the case was discussed in Ruth Hanley, In re T.A.C.P. *Issues in Law & Medicine* (1993): 9:1, 66.

39. *In the Matter of Baby K.* 832 F. Supp. 1022. (July 1993), 1027.

40. *In re T.A.C.P.* 609 So. 2d 588 (Fla. 1992), 589.

41. R. C. Lewontin, *Biology as Ideology* (New York: Harper Collins, 1993), 88.

42. Jürgen Habermas, *Justification and Application: Remarks on Discourse Ethics* (Cambridge, Mass.: MIT Press, 1993). Also see the use of "discourse ethics" in Post, *The Moral Challenge of Alzheimer Disease*, 17.

CHAPTER 2

An early version of this chapter is scheduled for publication as: Tom Koch, "Does the sanctity of human life doctrine sanctify humanness, or life?" *Cambridge Quarterly of Healthcare Ethics*, in press.

1. S. Bindeman, Judge stays on bench to fight his disease's "death sentence," *Toronto Star*, January 11, 1993, A1, 11.

2. Jenny M. Young, Carolyn L. Marshall, and Elizabeth J. Anderson, Amyotrophic lateral sclerosis patients' perspectives on use of mechanical ventilation, *Health and Social Work* (1994): 19:4, 253–60.

3. Ironically, Noel David Earley's electronic insistence on death rather than a restricted life was featured in a series by the *Providence (RI) Journal-Bulletin*, a newspaper whose continued employment and support of a columnist with advanced ALS was featured in the *American Journalism Review*. The Earley series was then placed on the Internet at Http://www.projo.com/special/noel/toc.htm. Also see Florence G. Graves, Writing for his life, *American Journalism Review* (March 1997): 25–31.

4. Sidney Callahan, Ethics and dementia: quality of life, *Alzheimer Disease and Associated Disorders* (1992): 6:3, 138.

5. Peter Singer, *Rethinking Life and Death: The Collapse of Our Traditional Ethics* (New York: St. Martin's Press, 1995), 1.

6. Margaret A. Somerville, Genetics, reproductive technologies, euthanasia, and the search for a new societal paradigm, *Social Science and Medicine* (1996): 42:12, ix–xii.

7. Joram Graf Haber, Review of Singer, Peter. Rethinking life and death, *Cambridge Quarterly of Healthcare Ethics* (1996).

8. James J. Hughes, Brain Death and Technological Change: Personal Identity, Neural Prostheses and Uploading, Second International Symposium on Brain Death, Havana, Cuba, February 27–March 1, 1995.

9. Ezekiel J. Emanuel, *The Ends of Human Life: Medical Ethics in a Liberal Polity* (Cambridge, Mass.: Harvard University Press, 1991), 11–13.

10. Kurt Bayertz, Techno-thanatology: Moral consequences of introducing brain criteria for death, *Journal of Medicine and Philosophy* (1992): 17, 407–17, quoted in J. Hughes, Brain death and technological change.

11. R. de Toedano, *Frontiers of Jazz*, 2d ed. (New York: Frederick Ungar Publishing, 1962), 71.

12. Philip R. Reilly, *The Surgical Solution: A History of Involuntary Sterilization in the United States* (Baltimore: John Hopkins University Press, 1991).

13. Martin S. Pernick, *The Black Stork: Eugenics and the Death of "Defective" Babies in American Medicine and Motion Pictures Since 1915* (New York: Oxford University Press, 1996), 3–18.

14. *Buck v Bell*, 274 US 200 (1927).

15. Stephen J. Gould, *The Mismeasure of Man* (New York: W. W. Norton, 1981), 335–36.

16. *Roe v Wade*, 410 US 113 (1973).

17. Gould, *The Mismeasure of Man*, 335–36.

18. Reilly, *The Surgical Solution*, 117.

19. S. E. Sytsma, Anencephalics as organ sources, *Theoretical Medicine* (1996): 17: 1, 19–32.

20. V. Burston, Breeding discontent, *Saturday Night* (June 1991): 15.

21. D. Goldhagen, *Hitler's Willing Executioners* (New York: Knopf, 1996), 119.

22. Pernick, *The Black Stork*, 163–64.

23. J. Horgan, Eugenics revisited, *Scientific American* (June 1993): 123.

24. S. J. Gould, The unkindest cut of all, in *Dinosaur in a Hay Stack* (New York: Harmony Books, 1995), 309–17.

25. Goldhagen, *Hitler's Willing Executioners*.

26. P. A. Byrne, J. C. Evers, and R. G. Niles, Anencephaly—Organ transplantation? *Issues in Law and Medicine* (1993): 9: 1, 23–33.

27. *In the Matter of Baby K* 832 F. Supp. 1022 (Va.: 9:1, 1993), 1029.

28. American Medical Association Council on Ethical and Judicial Affairs, The use of anencephalic neonates as organ donors, *Journal of the American Medical Association* (1995): 273: 20, 1614–18.

29. P. A. Byrne and R. G. Niles, The brain stem in brain death: A critical review, *Issues in Law and Medicine* (1993): 9: 1, 3–21.

30. *In re T.A.C.P.* 609 So. 2d 588 (Fla. 1992), 595.

31. See, for example, J. Lantos, Baby Doe five years later: Implications for child health, *New England Journal of Medicine* (1987): 317, 444–47; Evert Van Leeuwen and Gerrit K. Kimsma, Acting or letting go: Medical decision making in neonatology in the Netherlands, *Cambridge Quarterly of Healthcare Ethics* (1993): 2, 265–69.

32. Tom Koch, Normative and prescriptive criteria: The efficacy of organ transplantation allocation protocols, *Theoretical Medicine* (1996): 17: 1, 75–93.

33. Tom Koch, The Canadian question: What's so great about intelligence? *Cambridge Quarterly of Healthcare Ethics* (1996): 5: 2, 307–9.

34. For a discussion, see D. Callahan, *Setting Limits: Medical Goals in an Aging Society* (New York: Simon and Schuster, 1987).

35. Peter Singer, *Rethinking Life and Death* (New York: St. Martin's Press, 1995), 165.

36. C. Dunphy, For the love of a chimp, *Toronto Star*, April 26, 1996, B1.

37. R. Wright, *The Moral Animal* (New York: Pantheon Books, 1994).

38. J. M. Masson, *When Elephants Weep: The Emotional Lives of Animals* (New York: Delacorte Press, 1995).

39. At the June 1995 Bioethics Beyond Borders Conference in Berkeley, California, I asked a speaker advocating "New Reproductive Technologies" how he liked doing eugenics. Irritated, but attempting to be polite, he informed me that "we no longer call it that." Similarly, those advocating restricting medical care for the elderly insist it is not a eugenic policy but one based on cost efficiency.

40. See, for example, Lantos, Baby Doe five years later.

41. Margaret A. Somerville, Genetics, reproductive technologies, euthanasia,

and the search for a new societal paradigm, *Social Science and Medicine* (1996): 42: 12, ix–xii.

42. Stephen G. Post, *The Moral Challenge of Alzheimer Disease* (Baltimore: Johns Hopkins University Press, 1995), 95.

43. J. R. Bach and D. I. Campangolo, Psychosocial adjustment of post-poliomyelitis ventilator assisted individuals, *Archives of Physical Medicine and Rehabilitation* (1992): 934–39.

44. Dickinson quoted in Florence George Graves, Writing for his life, *American Journalism Review* (March 1997): 30.

45. K. A. Gerhart et al., Quality of life following spinal cord injury: Knowledge and attitudes of emergency care providers, *Annals of Emergency Medicine* (1994): 23: 4, 807–12.

46. Jenny M. Young, Carolyn L. Marshall, and Elizabeth J. Anderson, Amyotrophic lateral sclerosis patients' perspectives on use of mechanical ventilation, *Health and Social Work* (1994): 19: 4, 253–60.

47. Jean-Dominique Bauby, *The Diving-Bell & the Butterfly* (London: Fourth Estate Limited, 1997).

48. See, for example, Karen S. Schneider and Jane Shapiro, Local hero, *People Magazine*, January 27, 1997, 82–86. For Reeve's own account, see Christopher Reeve, *Still Me: A Life* (New York: Random House, 1998).

49. Jenny M. Young and Paule McNicoll, Against all odds: Positive life experiences of persons with advanced amyotrophic lateral sclerosis, *Health and Social Work* (1998): 23: 1, 35–43.

50. Helga Kuhse and Peter Singer, *Should the Baby Live? The Problem of Handicapped Infants* (Oxford: Oxford University Press, 1985), 143.

51. J. Glover, *Causing Death and Saving Lives* (Harmondsworth, England: Penguin, 1977), 52–53, quoted in Paula Boddington and Tessa Podpadec, Measuring quality of life in theory and in practice: A dialogue between philosophical and psychological approaches, *Bioethics* (1992): 6:3, 202–17.

52. D. W. Brock, *Life and Death: Philosophical Essays in Medical Bioethics* (New York: Cambridge University Press, 1993), 372, quoted in Post, *Moral Challenge.*

53. See, for example, Tom Koch, *A Place in Time: Care Givers for Their Elderly* (Westport, Conn.: Praeger, 1993).

54. Karl Binding and A. Hoche, Permitting the destruction of unworthy life: Its extent and form, Walter Wright, trans., *Issues in Law and Medicine* (1992): 8: 2, 231–65.

55. Daniel Callahan, *Setting Limits: Medical Goals for an Aging Society* (New York: Simon and Schuster, 1987).

56. James W. Walters, Proximate personhood as a standard for making difficult treatment decisions: Imperiled newborns as a case study, *Bioethics* (1992): 6:1, 12–22.

57. J. Harris, *The Value of Life* (London: Routledge, 1985), also quoted in

David P. Price, Contemporary transplant initiatives: Where's the harm in them? *Journal of Law, Medicine & Ethics* (1996): 24:2, 242.

58. Dave Thomasma, Anencephalics as organ donors, *Biomedical Ethics Reviews—1989*, ed. James M. Humber and Robert F. Almeder (Clifton, N.J.: Humana Press, 1990), 25–54.

59. Walters, Proximate personhood as a standard for making difficult treatment decisions, 12–22.

60. Post, *Moral Challenge*, 108.

61. Oliver Sacks, The lost mariner, in *The Man Who Mistook His Wife for a Hat* (New York: Summit Books, 1985), 22–41.

62. Oliver Sacks, *Awakenings* (1973; London: Pan Books, 1982).

CHAPTER 3

1. Amy Gutmann and Dennis Thompson, *Democracy and Disagreement* (Cambridge, Mass.: Harvard University Press, 1996), 35.

2. John Rawls, *Political Liberalism* (New York: Columbia University Press, 1993), 229, quoted in Amy Gutmann and Dennis Thompson, *Democracy and Disagreement* (Cambridge, Mass.: Harvard University Press, 1996), 36.

3. W. B. Gallie, Essentially contestible concepts, *Proceedings of the Aristotelian Society* (1955): 56. I am obliged to Donald Ainslie, philosophy professor at the University of Toronto, for this citation and for his discussion of the issues involved.

4. Timothy E. Quill and Gerrit Kimsma, End-of-life care in the Netherlands and the United States: A comparison of values, justifications, and practices, *Cambridge Quarterly of Healthcare Ethics* (1997): 6:2, 189–204.

5. Robert Audi, ed., *The Cambridge Dictionary of Philosophy* (New York: Cambridge University Press, 1995).

6. Jeremy Brown, Research on human embryos—A justification, *Journal of Medical Ethics* (1986): 12:4, 201–5. Brown argues that life begins and ends with evidence of pulse and respiration and with the capacity for consciousness and sentience.

7. John Goldenring, The brain-life theory: Towards a consistent biological definition of humanness, *Journal of Medical Ethics* (1985): 11:2, 198–204.

8. J. A. Burges and S. A. Tawia, When did you first begin to feel it? Locating the beginning of human consciousness, *Bioethics* (1996): 6:1, 3–14.

9. Harold J. Morowitz, *The Facts of Life: Science & the Abortion Controversy* (New York: Oxford University Press, 1992).

10. James J. Hughes, Brain Death and Technological Change: Personal Identity, Neural Prostheses, and Uploading, Second International Symposium on Brain Death, Havana, Cuba, February 27–March 1, 1995.

11. Jeffery Spike and Jane Greenlaw, Ethics consultation: Persistent brain

death and religion: Must a person believe in death to die? *Journal of Law, Medicine and Ethics* (1995): 23:3, 20–23.

12. Paul A. Byrne and Richard G. Niles, The brain stem in brain death: A critical review, *Issues in Law and Medicine* (1993): 9:1, 3–21.

13. *In re T.A.C.P.* 609 So. 2d 588 (Fla. 1992). The case resulted in a flood of popular and technical articles. See, for example, Ruth A. Hanley, *In re T.A.C.P.*, *Issues in Law and Medicine* (1993): 9:1, 65–68.

14. *In the Matter of Baby K* 832 F. Supp. 1022 (Va. 1993), 1027.

15. Susan M. Wolf, Shifting paradigms in bioethics and health law: The rise of a new pragmatism, *American Journal of Law and Medicine* (1994): 20:4, 395–415.

16. Raanan Gillon, Transplantation and ethics, in *Birth to Death: Science and Ethics*, ed. David Thomasma and Thomasine Kushner (New York: Cambridge University Press, 1996), 106–18.

17. T. L. Beauchamp and J. F. Childress, *Principles of Biomedical Ethics*, 4th ed. (New York: Oxford University Press, 1994).

18. Gillon, Transplantation and ethics, 106–18.

19. Loren E. Lomasky, *Persons, Rights, and the Moral Community* (New York: Oxford University Press, 1987), 11.

20. John Rawls, *A Theory of Justice* (Cambridge, Mass.: Harvard University Press, 1971).

21. See, in the area of social debate, Eva F. Kittay and Diana T. Meyers, The justice position and the care perspective, in *Women and Moral Theory*, ed. Eva F. Kittay and Diana T. Meyers (Savage, Md. Rowman and Littlefield, 1987), 4–10.

22. Charles Taylor, *The Ethics of Authenticity* (Cambridge, Mass.: Harvard University Press, 1992).

23. Oliver Sacks, *Awakenings* (1973; London: Pan Books, 1982), 238–39.

24. Laurence H. Tribe, *Abortion: The Clash of Absolutes* (New York: W. W. Norton, 1990), 5.

25. Tom Koch, Normative and prescriptive criteria: The efficacy of organ transplantation allocation protocols, *Theoretical Medicine* (1996): 17:1, 75–93.

26. Ronald Dworkin, *Taking Rights Seriously* (Cambridge, Mass.: Harvard University Press, 1978).

27. E. H. Morreim, *Balancing Act: The New Medical Ethics of Medicine's New Economics* (Dodrecht and Boston: Kluwer Academic Publications, 1991), 85, quoted in Mark J. Bilton and Stuart G. Ginder, The eclipse of the individual in policy (Where is the place for justice?), *Cambridge Quarterly of Healthcare Ethics* (1996): 5:4, 528.

28. Thomas L. Saaty, *The Analytic Hierarchy Process* (New York: McGraw-Hill, 1980); L. Thomas Saaty, *Fundamentals of Decision Making and Priority Theory with the Analytic Hierarchy Process* (Pittsburgh: RWS Publications, 1994).

29. D. Olson, *Decision Aids for Selection Problems* (New York: Springer-Verlag, 1996).

30. Thomas L. Saaty and Luis G. Vargas, *Decision Making in Economic, Political, Social and Technological Environments*. AHP Series Vol. 7 (Pittsburgh, PA: RWS Publications, 1994).

31. I. Basak and T. Saaty, Group decision making using the Analytic Hierarchy Process, *Journal of Mathematical Modeling* (1993): 17, 415.

32. Thomas L. Saaty and Joyce M. Alexander, *Conflict Resolution: The Analytic Hierarchy Process* (New York: Praeger, 1989).

33. Alan D. Taylor, *Mathematics and Politics: Strategy, Voting, Power, and Proof* (New York: Springer-Verlag, 1997), 242–45.

CHAPTER 4

An earlier version of this chapter appeared as Tom Koch, Normative and prescriptive criteria: The efficacy of organ transplantation allocation protocols, *Theoretical Medicine* (1996): 17:1, 75–93.

1. Files of the following newspapers were searched in preparation for this chapter: *Calgary Herald, Vancouver Sun, Toronto Star, Ottawa Citizen, Edmonton Journal*. All are collected and indexed daily on both Informart/Dialogue (file 727) and on Dow Jones News Retrieval ("Canadian Newspapers").

2. Chris Dawson, Supporters rally for teen's transplant, *Calgary Herald*, March 28, 1995, B3.

3. Darcy Henton, "Wasted" transplants under fire in Alberta, *Toronto Star*, April 7, 1995, A10.

4. Hearts needed, *Toronto Star*, April 18, 1995, A20.

5. Child a human being, *Calgary Herald*, April 23, 1995, A7.

6. Health service trying to play God, *Calgary Herald*, April 13, 1995, A6.

7. Tom Donohue, Morally outrageous, *Ottawa Citizen*, March 22, 1995, A12.

8. Henton, "Wasted" transplants.

9. Ibid.

10. Ibid.

11. Ibid.

12. Transplant rules revised, *Edmonton Journal*, April 5, 1995, B2.

13. Organ transplantation is a basic medical service covered under the Canada Health Act. Individual provinces administer organ transplant programs which, like health care itself, are under the general jurisdiction of provincial health ministries. Thus, in Canada questions of third-party insurance and the cost of transplant procedures is not an issue.

14. M. E. Olbrisch and J. L. Levenson, Psychosocial evaluation of heart transplant candidates: An international survey of process, criteria, and outcomes, *Journal of Heart Lung Transplant* (1991): 10, 948–55, quoted in Rachel A. Majeske, Criteria for transplant candidate Selection, *BIOMED-L. Conference List*, Internet, August 16, 1995.

15. Gary Delsohn and Tom Philip, Activist takes on fight for her life, *Sacramento Bee*, August 11, 1995, A1.

16. Ibid.

17. Sabin Russell, Livers for transplant can show up quickly, *San Francisco Chronicle*, June 9, 1995, A6.

18. Michael Miller, Reuters News Service (America Online: TVnewsnut), August 27, 1995.

19. Arthur Hoppe, Mickey Mantle's lucky liver, *San Francisco Chronicle*, June 16, 1995, A29.

20. Interview with Dr. Arthur Caplan, "All Things Considered," Canadian Broadcasting Corporation, June 7, 1995.

21. Hoppe, Mickey Mantle's lucky liver. The original statement appeared in Gina Kolata, Transplants, morality and Mickey Mantle, *New York Times*, June 11, 1995.

22. Ibid.

23. Martin, Benjamin, Carl Cohen, and Eugence Grochowski, What transplantation can teach us about health care reform, *New England Journal of Medicine* (1994): 330:12, 858–60.

24. Current proponents of health care rationing, for example, typically assume a context of relative scarcity. See, for example, Daniel Callahan, *Setting Limits: Medical Goals in an Aging Society* (New York: Simon and Schuster, 1987).

25. See, for example, Jacqueline J. Glover and Cindy H. Rushton, From Baby Doe to Baby K: Evolving challenges in pediatric ethics, *Journal of Law, Medicine & Ethics* (1995): 23:1, 5–6; John Lantos, Baby Doe five years later: Implications for child health, *New England Journal of Medicine* (1987): 317, 444–47; G. Y. York, R. M. Ballarno, and R. O. York, Baby Doe regulations and medical judgment, *Social Science and Medicine* (1990): 30, 654–67.

26. In debate on U.S. federal support for universal dialysis, Indiana Senator Vance Hartke told the U.S. Congress that a society able to afford billions of dollars annually on cosmetics and other nonessential items, *should* "set our national priorities through a national effort to bring kidney disease treatment within reach of all those in need," *Congressional Record*, September 30, 1972, 33,004–33,008. Since that debate, the approximately $3 billion annual cost for dialysis treatment for 150,000 U.S. patients has been federally funded.

27. UNOS Scientific Registry, July 9, 1995. UNOS statistics are updated periodically and available through a variety of venues including online at http://www.unos.org/.

28. Benjamin, Cohen, and Grochowski, 859.

29. Helga Kuhse defines the principle: "It is absolutely prohibited either intentionally to kill a patient or intentionally to let a patient die, and to base decisions relating to prolongation or shortening of human life on considerations of quality or kind," quoted in Stephen G. Post, Baby K: Medical futility and the free exercise of religion, *Journal of Law, Medicine & Ethics* (1995): 23:1, 21.

30. T. E. Startzl et al., Equitable allocation of extrarenal organs: With special reference to the liver, *Transplantation Proceedings* (1988): 20:1, 131–38.

31. Thomas E. Starzl et al., A multifactorial system for equitable selection of cadaver kidney recipients, *Journal of the American Medical Association* (1987): 257: 22, 3073–75.

32. Startzl, Equitable allocation of extra renal organs, 133.

33. UNOS Scientific Registry, April 6, 1995.

34. D. R. Cook et al., A method to allocate livers for orthotopic transplantation: An application of the Analytic Hierarchy Process, *Proceedings of the International Conference on Multiple Criteria Decision Making Applications in Industry and Service*, Asian Institute of Technology, Bangkok, December 6–8, 1989; UNOS, *The Feasibility of Allocating Organs on the Basis of a Single National List* (Richmond: National Organ Procurement and Transplantation Network, December 1991), 6–7.

35. Cook, A method to allocate livers.

36. UNOS, *The Feasibility of Allocating Organs*, 6–7.

37. At present, the maximum acceptable preservation time is four hours for heart, lung, and heart-lung transplants, eight to ten hours for pancreatic and liver transplants, and thirty-six hours for kidney transplants. Paul J. Hauptman and Kevin J. O'Connor, Medical progress: Procurement and allocation of solid organs for transplantation, *New England Journal of Medicine* (February 6, 1997): 226:6, 422–431.

38. Startzl et al., Equitable allocation of extra renal organs, 133.

39. Ibid., 131.

40. Cook, A method to allocate livers, 782.

41. Gloria J. Banks, Legal and ethical safeguards: Protection of society's most vulnerable participants in a commercialized organ transplantation system, *American Journal of Law and Medicine* (1995): 21:1, 2.

42. Ibid., 92.

43. See for example Lawrence Gottlieb and Mark J. Zucker, Organs for undocumented aliens? A transplantation dilemma, *Cambridge Quarterly of Healthcare Ethics* (1995): 4:2, 231. At Newark (N.J.) Beth Israel Medical Center. "The individual must be evaluated and accepted in accordance with all appropriate clinical standards . . . including psychosocial compatibility."

44. Gregory S. Crespi, Overcoming the legal obstacles to the creation of a futures market in bodily organs, *Ohio State Law Journal* (1994): 55, 14–15.

45. Henry S. Perkins, Commentary: Distributing American hearts for transplantation: The predicament of living in the global village, *Cambridge Quarterly of Healthcare Ethics* (1995): 4:2, 232–36.

46. See, for example, Banks, Legal and ethical safeguards, 63–64.

47. Henton, "Wasted" transplants, A10.

48. S. Tesh, *Hidden Arguments: Political Ideology and Disease Prevention Policy* (New Brunswick, N.J.: Rutgers University Press, 1988) 34, quoted in Max

Charlesworth, *Bioethics in a Liberal Society* (New York: Cambridge University Press, 1993), 119.

49. W. Edwards, and B. F. Hutton, Smarts and SMARTER: Improved simple methods for multiattribute utility measurements, *Organizational Behavior and Human Decision Process* (1994): 60, 311.

50. Martin S. Pernick, *The Black Stork: Eugenics and the Death of "Defective" Babies in American Medicine and Motion Pictures Since 1915* (New York: Oxford University Press, 1995), 71.

51. Olbrisch and Levenson, Psychosocial evaluation of heart transplant candidates, 948–55.

52. C. West Churchman, *A Systems Approach*, rev. ed. (New York: Dell, 1979), 139–41.

53. M. C. Corley and G. Sneed, Criteria in the selection of organ transplant recipients, *Heart and Lung* (1994): 23, 446–57, quoted in Rachel A. Majeske, Criteria for transplant candidate selection, *BIOMED-L. Conference List*, Internet, August 16, 1995.

54. Delsohn and Philip, Activist takes on fight for her life.

CHAPTER 5

A preliminary report of the hospital group's responses appeared as Tom Koch and M. Rowell, A pilot study on transplant eligibility criteria: Valuing the stories in numbers, *Pediatric Nursing* (1997): 23:2, 160–66.

1. Nicholas Rescher, *Pluralism: Against the Demand for Consensus* (New York: Oxford University Press, 1995), 185.

2. Jonathan D. Moreno, *Deciding Together: Bioethics and Moral Consensus* (New York: Oxford University Press, 1995).

3. Mark Kuczewski, Review of Jonathan D. Moreno, *Deciding Together: Bioethics and Moral Consensus*, *Cambridge Quarterly of Healthcare Ethics* (1997): 6:3, 358–59.

4. Rescher *Pluralism*, 185.

5. Barbara B. Ott, Commentary on Tom Koch and M. Rowell, Changes in liver transplantation policy, *Pediatric Nursing* (1997): 23:2, 167–68.

6. G. Kolata, In shift, prospects for survival will decide liver transplants, *New York Times*, November 15, 1996, A1, A26; R. Estrin, Liver transplant policy to favor patients most likely to survive, *Washington Post*, November 15, 1996, A3; also quoted in Ott, Changes in liver transplantation policy.

7. Ott, changes in liver transplantation policy.

8. Gina Kolata, Transplants, morality, and Mickey Mantle, *New York Times*, June 11, 1995, Section 4, 5.

9. Gary Delsohn and Tom Philip, Activist takes on fight for her life: Transplant rejected because of disability, *Sacramento Bee*, August 11, 1995, A1.

10. Tom Koch, The Canadian question: What's so great about intelligence? *Cambridge Quarterly of Healthcare Ethics* (1996): 5:2, 307–10.

11. Cynthia Hubert, Transplant pioneer loses battle for life, *Sacramento Bee*, May 25, 1997.

12. T. E. Startzl et al., Equitable allocation of extrarenal organs: With special reference to the liver, *Transplantation Proceedings* (1988): 20:1, 131–38.

13. Michelle Oberman, Minor rights and wrongs, *Journal of Law, Medicine & Ethics* (1996): 24:2, 127–38.

14. E. L. Ramos et al., The evaluation of candidates for renal transplantation: The current practice of U.S. transplant centers, *Transplantation* (1994): 57, 490–97.

15. A. Giangrande, How to assess the weights of the criteria in the AHP, Presented at the Fourth IAHP Conference, Simon Fraser University, Burnaby, B.C., July 1996. Also see, Thomas L. Saaty, An exposition of the AHP to the paper, "Remarks on the Analytic Hierarchy Process," *Management Science* (1990): 36, 259–68.

16. M. C. Corley and G. Sneed, Criteria in the selection of organ transplant recipients, *Heart and Lung* (1994): 23:6, 453–454.

17. R. S. Osorio et al., Predicting recidivism after orthotopic liver transplantation for alcoholic liver disease, *Hematology* (1994): 20:1, 105–10.

18. Andrew Jameton *Nursing Practice: The Ethical Issues* (Englewood Cliffs, N.J.: Prentice Hall, 1984), 24, quoted in Daniel F. Chambliss, *Beyond Caring: Hospitals, Nurses, and the Social Organization of Ethics* (Chicago: University of Chicago Press, 1996), 138.

19. Chambliss, *Beyond Caring*.

20. Margaret Somerville, Euthanasia by confusion, *UNSW Law Journal* (1997): 23:3, 1–20.

21. Chambliss, *Beyond Caring*.

CHAPTER 6

An earlier version of this chapter appeared as Tom Koch and Mark Ridgley, Aids, anencephaly, and AHP, *Proceedings of the Fourth International Symposium on the Analytic Hierarchy Process*, Burnaby, B. C., July 12–15, 1996, 363–73. The approach was also described in Tom Koch and Mark Ridgley, Distance perspectives: Aids, anencephaly, and AHP, *Theoretical Medicine and Bioethics* (1998): 19: 1, 47–58.

1. *In the Matter of Baby K*. 832 F. Supp. 1022. (Va. 1993), 1027.

2. *In re T.A.C.P.* 609 So. 2d 588 (Fla. 1992), 589.

3. See, for example, P. A. Byrne, J. C. Evers, and R. G. Niles, Anencephaly—Organ transplantation? *Issues in Law and Medicine* (1993): 9:1, 23–33; Jacqueline J. Glover and Cindy H. Rushton, From Baby Doe to Baby K: Evolving challenges in pediatric ethics, *Journal of Law, Medicine & Ethics* (1995): 23:1, 5–

67; A. B. Goldberg, *In the matter of Baby K*, Letters to the Editor, *Journal of Law, Medicine & Ethics* (1995): 23:3, 300.

4. B. Spielman, Collective decisions about medical futility, *Journal of Law, Medicine & Ethics* (1995): 22:2, 152–60.

5. J. McKnight, Two tools for well-being: Health systems and communities, *Annals of Preventive Medicine*, Supplement: *Medicine in the 21st Century: Challenges in Personal and Public Health Promotion* (1994): 10:3, 23–26.

6. Eva F. Kittay and Diana T. Meyers, The justice position and the care perspective, in *Women and Moral Theory*, ed. Eva F. Kittay and Diana T. Meyers (Savage, Md.: Rowman and Littlefield, 1987), 4–10.

7. D. W. Brock, Voluntary active euthanasia, in *Dying Well? A Colloquy on Euthanasia & Assisted Suicide*, *Hastings Center Report* (1992): 22:2, 11. Howard Brody, Assisted death—A compassionate response to medical failure, *New England Journal of Medicine* (1992): 327, 124–28.

8. J. Harris, *The Value of Life* (London: Routledge, 1985), 242.

9. Judith F. Darr, Medical futility and implications for physician autonomy, *American Journal of Law and Medicine* (1995) 21:2–3, 223.

10. R. A. Hanley, *In re T.A.C.P.*, *Issues in Law and Medicine* (1993): 9:1, 67.

11. D. Dennet, Conditions of personhood, in A. R. Oksenberg, *The Identities of Persons* (Berkeley: University of California Press, 1975), 175.

12. J. Fletcher, *Humanhood: Essays in Biomedical Ethics* (Buffalo, N.Y.: Prometheus Books, 1979), 7–19.

13. R. Rymer, A silent childhood, II, *New Yorker*, April 20, 1992, 67–69.

14. D. Rabiner and J. Coie, Effect of expectancy indications on rejected children's acceptance by unfamiliar peers, *Developmental Psychology* (1989): 25, 450–57; Rosenbaum P. L. and R. W. Armstrong, Self-perceived social function among disabled children in regular classrooms, *Developmental and Behavioral Pediatrics* (1992): 13.1, 11–16; A. Lefebvre and E. Arndt, Working with facially disfigured children: A challenge in prevention, *Canadian Journal of Psychiatry* (1988): 33.

15. P. A. Byrne and R. G. Niles, The brain stem in brain death: A critical review, *Issues in Law and Medicine* (1993): 9:1, 3–21.

16. L. J. Silberstein, *Martin Buber's Social and Religious Thought* (New York: New York University Press, 1989), 128.

17. The social meaning of such cases has been a theme in the work of Oliver Sacks. See, for example, *An Anthropologist on Mars* (New York: Knopf, 1995); *The Man Who Mistook His Wife for a Hat* (New York: Summit, 1985).

18. Lewis Thomas, *The Fragile Species* (New York: Collier Books, 1992), 26.

19. The complex interrelation of time and memory to personality has been reviewed recently by Sacks, *An Anthropologist on Mars*, chapters 2 and 4.

20. See, for example, Hilde L. Nelson, Dethroning choice: Analogy, personhood, and the new reproductive technologies, *Journal of Law, Medicine & Ethics* (1995): 23:2, 133–34, Silberstein, *Martin Buber's Social and Religious Thought*.

21. For example, Daniel Callahan, *Setting Limits: Medical Goals in an Aging*

Society (New York: Simon and Schuster, 1987). In allocating health care resources, Callahan emphasizes youth's future potential while devaluing the past contribution of older citizens.

22. "Fair innings" is an argument used by some advocating disadvantaging seniors in allocative schemes because they've had their "fair innings" and scarce social resources and thus should be used to assure younger persons have a similar opportunity.

23. Martin R. Cohn, Defiant Rabin assassin jailed for life, *Toronto Star*, February 28, 1996, A20.

24. Michael Fleeman, His face a stone as jury seals fate, *Toronto Star*, June 14, 1997, A1.

25. Sacks; *An Anthropologist on Mars*, 275–76.

26. See, for example, Isaac Asimov and Robert Silverberg, *The Positronic Man* (New York: Doubleday, 1993).

27. John Lantos, Baby Doe five years later: Implications for child health, *New England Journal of Medicine* (1987); 317, 444–47; G. Y. York, R. M. Balarno, and R. O. York, Baby Doe regulations and medical judgment, *Social Science and Medicine* (1990): 30, 657–64.

28. See, for example, Jacqueline J. Glover and Cindy H. Rushton, From Baby Doe to Baby K: Evolving challenges in pediatric ethics, *Journal of Law, Medicine & Ethics* (1995): 23:1, 5–6.

29. John Hardwig, What about the family? *Hastings Center Report* (1990): 20: 2, 5–10.

30. Oliver Sacks, *Awakenings* (1973; London: Pan Books, 1982), 238–39.

31. Lawrence J. Schneiderman and Sharyn Manning, *The Baby K Case*: A search for the elusive standard of medical care, *Cambridge Quarterly of Healthcare Ethics* (1997): 6:1, 9–18.

32. Ibid., 13–14.

33. Sacks, *Awakenings*, 251.

34. Ibid.

CHAPTER 7

1. James L. Nelson, Taking families seriously, *Hastings Center Report* (1992): 22:4, 6–12.

2. David Raphael, *Moral Philosophy* (Oxford: Oxford University Press, 1981), 1.

3. Nelson, *Taking families seriously*, 7.

4. Mildred Z. Solomon, From what's neutral to what's meaningful: Reflections on a study of medical interpreters, *The Journal of Clinical Ethics* (1997): 8: 1, 88–93.

5. Albert R. Jonsen, Casuistry: An alternative or complement to principles? *Kennedy Institute of Ethics Journal* (1995): 5:3, 237–51.

6. Susan M. Wolf, Shifting paradigms in bioethics and health law: The rise of a new pragmatism, *American Journal of Law and Medicine* (1994): 20:4, 395–415.

7. G. L. Wackers, *Constructivist Medicine* (Maastricht, Holland: Universitaire Pers Maastricht, 1994).

8. Jürgen Habermas, *Justification and Application: Remarks on Discourse Ethics* (Cambridge, Mass.: MIT Press, 1993). See also its application by Stephen G. Post, *The Moral Challenge of Alzheimer Disease* (Baltimore: Johns Hopkins University Press, 1995).

9. Martha Minow and Elizabeth V. Spelman, In context 63, *Southern California Law Review* (1990): 1597, 1632–33, quoted in Wolf, Shifting paradigms, 413.

10. Michael Walzer, *Thick and Thin: Moral Argument at Home and Abroad* (Notre Dame, Ind.: Notre Dame University Press, 1994), 4.

11. I am obliged to Donald C. Ainslie, University of Toronto, Department of Philosophy for this observation, and earlier, for his reading of a draft of chapter 3.

12. Raanan Gillon, *Philosophical Medical Ethics* (Chichester, England: John Wiley and Sons, 1985), 2.

13. Thomas L. Beauchamp and J. F. Childress, *Principles of Bioethics*, 4th ed. (New York: Oxford University Press, 1994), 3.

14. Donald C. Ainslie, AIDS, sexual ethics, and the duty to warn: Expanding the boundaries of bioethics. Unpublished paper, 1997.

15. Harvey D. Klevit et al., Prioritization of health care services: A progress report by the Oregon Health Services Commission, *Archives of Internal Medicine* (1991): 151, 912–16.

16. Robert M. Veatch, Research on "big ticket" items: Ethical implications for equitable access, *Journal of Law, Medicine & Ethics* (1994): 22:2, 148–51.

17. Robert M. Veatch, Should basic care get priority? Doubts about rationing the Oregon way, *Kennedy Institute of Ethics Journal* (1991): 1:3, 187–206.

18. Veatch, Research on "big ticket" items, 151.

19. Roger Crisp, Tony Hope, and David Ebbs, The Asbury draft policy on ethical use of resources, *British Medical Journal* (1996): 312:7045, 1528–31.

20. Ibid.

21. Peter Dormer, Commentary: Courageous attempt, but needs clarification, commentary on the Asbury draft policy, *British Medical Journal* (1996): 312:7045, 1532.

22. Dave Thomasma, Commentary: Guidelines for rationing resemble process of family decision making, commentary on the Asbury draft policy, *British Medical Journal* (1996): 312:7045, 1531–32.

23. Gina Kolata, Transplants, morality, and Mickey Mantle, *New York Times*, June 11, 1995, Section 4, 5.

Bibliography

Ainslie, Donald C. AIDS, sexual ethics, and the duty to warn: Expanding the boundaries of bioethics. Unpublished paper, 1997.

Alexander, Shana. They decide who lives, who dies. *Life Magazine*, November 9, 1962.

American Medical Association Council on Ethical and Judicial Affairs. The use of anencephalic neonates as organ donors. *Journal of the American Medicine Association* (1995): 273: 20, 1614–18.

Asimov, Isaac, and Robert Silverberg. *The Positronic Man*. New York: Doubleday, 1993.

Audi, Robert, ed. *The Cambridge Dictionary of Philosophy*. New York: Cambridge University Press, 1995.

Bach, J. R., and D. I. Campangolo. Psychosocial adjustment of post–poliomyelitis ventilator assisted individuals. *Archives of Physical Medicine and Rehabilitation* (1992): 934–39.

Banks, Gloria J. Legal and ethical safeguards: Protection of society's most vulnerable participants in a commercialized organ transplantation system. *American Journal of Law and Medicine* (1995): 21: 1, 45–110.

Basak, I., and T. Saaty. Group decision making using the Analytic Hierarchy Process. *Journal of Mathematical Modeling* (1993): 17, 415.

Bauby, Jean-Dominique. *The Diving-Bell & the Butterfly*. London: Fourth Estate Limited, 1997.

Bayertz, Kurt. Techno-thanatology: Moral consequences of introducing brain criteria for death. *Journal of Medicine and Philosophy* (1992): 17, 407–17.

Beauchamp, T. L., and J. F. Childress. *Principles of Biomedical Ethics*. 4th ed. New York: Oxford University Press, 1994.

Benjamin, M., C. Cohen, and E. Grochowski. What transplantation can teach us about health care reform. *New England Journal of Medicine* (1994): 330: 12, 858–60.

Bilton, Mark J., and Stuart G. Ginder. The eclipse of the individual in policy (Where is the place for justice?). *Cambridge Quarterly of Healthcare Ethics* (1996): 5:4, 528.

Bindeman, S. Judge stays on bench to fight his disease's "death sentence." *Toronto Star*, January 11, 1993, A1, 11.

Binding, Karl, and A. Hoche. Permitting the destruction of unworthy life: Its extent and form. Trans. Walter Wright. *Issues in Law and Medicine* (1992): 8:2, 231–65.

Boddington, Paula, and Tessa Podpadec. Measuring quality of life in theory and in practice: A dialogue between philosophical and psychological approaches. *Bioethics* (1992): 6:3, 202–17.

Brock, D. W. *Life and Death: Philosophical Essays in Medical Bioethics.* New York: Cambridge University Press, 1993.

Brock, D. W. Voluntary active euthanasia. *Dying Well? A Colloquy on Euthanasia & Assisted Suicide.* Hastings Center Report (1992): 22:2, 11.

Brody, Howard. Assisted death—A compassionate response to medical failure. *New England Journal of Medicine* (1992): 327, 124–28.

Brown, Jeremy. Research on human embryos—A justification. *Journal of Medical Ethics* (1986): 12:4, 201–5.

Buck v Bell, 274 US 200 (1927).

Burges, J. A., and S. A. Tawia. When did you first begin to feel it? Locating the beginning of human consciousness. *Bioethics* (1996): 6:1, 3–14.

Burston, V. Breeding discontent. *Saturday Night* (June 1991): 15.

Byrne, P. A., J. C. Evers, and R. G. Niles. Anencephaly—Organ transplantation? *Issues in Law and Medicine* (1993): 9:1, 23–33.

Byrne, P. A., and R. G. Niles. The brain stem in brain death: A critical review. *Issues in Law and Medicine* (1993): 9:1, 3–21.

Callahan, Daniel. *Setting Limits: Medical Goals in an Aging Society.* New York: Simon and Schuster, 1987.

Callahan, Sidney. Ethics and dementia: Quality of life. *Alzheimer Disease and Associated Disorders* (1992): 6:3, 138–44.

Caplan, Arthur L. What bioethics brought to the public. *Hastings Center Report,* Special Supplement (November/December 1993): S14–S15.

Chambliss, Daniel F. *Beyond Caring: Hospitals, Nurses, and the Social Organization of Ethics.* Chicago: University of Chicago Press, 1996.

Charlesworth, Max. *Bioethics in a Liberal Society.* New York: Cambridge University Press, 1993.

Churchman, C. West. *A Systems Approach.* Rev. ed. New York: Dell, 1979.

Congressional Record. September 30, 1972; 33,004–33,008.

Cook, D., et al. A method to allocate livers for orthotopic transplantation: An application of the Analytic Hierarchy Process. *Proceedings of the Interna-*

tional Conference on Multiple Criteria Decision Making Applications in Industry and Service. Asian Institute of Technology, Bangkok, December 6–8, 1989.

Corley, M. C., and G. Sneed. Criteria in the selection of organ transplant Recipients. *Heart and Lung* (1994): 23:6, 446–57.

Crespi, Gregory S. Overcoming the legal obstacles to the creation of a futures market in bodily organs. *Ohio State Law Journal* (1994): 55, 14–15.

Crisp, Roger, Tony Hope, and David Ebbs. The Asbury draft policy on ethical use of resources. *British Medical Journal* (1996): 312:7045, 1528–31.

Darr, Judith F. Medical futility and implications for physician autonomy. *American Journal of Law and Medicine* (1995): 21: 2–3, 223.

Dawson, Chris. Supporters rally for teen's transplant. *Calgary Herald*, March 28, 1995, B3.

Delsohn, Gary, and Tom Philip. Activist takes on fight for her life. *Sacramento Bee*, August 11, 1995, A1.

de Toedano, R. *Frontiers of Jazz.* 2d ed. New York: Frederick Ungar Publishing, 1962.

Dennet, D. Conditions of personhood. In *The Identities of Persons*, ed. A. R. Oksenberg. Berkeley: University of California Press, 1975, 175.

Donohue, Tom. Morally outrageous. *Ottawa Citizen*, March 22, 1995, A12.

Dormer, Peter. Commentary: Courageous attempt, but needs clarification. Commentary on the Asbury draft policy. *British Medical Journal* (1996): 312: 7045, 1532.

Dunphy, C. For the love of chimps. *Toronto Star*, April 26, 1996, B1.

Dworkin, Ronald. *Taking Rights Seriously.* Cambridge, Mass.: Harvard University Press, 1978.

Edwards, W., and B. F. Hutton. Smarts and SMARTER: Improved simple methods for multiattribute utility measurements. *Organizational Behavior and Human Decision Process* (1994): 60, 311.

Emanuel, Ezekiel J. *The Ends of Human Life: Medical Ethics in a Liberal Polity.* Cambridge, Mass.: Harvard University Press, 1991.

Estrin, R. Liver transplant policy to favor patients most likely to survive. *Washington Post*, November 15, 1996, A3.

Fernandez, Abel A. Expert choice: Software review. *OR/MS Today* (Online Edition) (1996): 23:4.

Fletcher, J. *Humanhood: Essays in Biomedical Ethics.* Buffalo, N.Y.: Prometheus Books, 1979.

Gallie, W. B. Essentially contestable concepts. *Proceedings of the Aristotelian Society* (1955): 56.

Gerhart, K. A., J. Koziol-McLain, S. R. Lowenstein, and G. Whiteneck. Quality of life following spinal cord injury: Knowledge and attitudes of emergency care providers. *Annals of Emergency Medicine* (1994): 23:4, 807–12.

Giangrande, A. How to assess the weights of the criteria in the AHP. Presented at the Fourth IAHP Conference, Simon Fraser University, Burnaby, B.C., July 1996.

Gillon, Raanan. Transplantation and ethics. In *Birth to Death: Science and Ethics*, ed. David Thomasma and Thomasine Kushner. New York: Cambridge University Press, 1996.

———. *Philosophical Medical Ethics*. Chichester, England: John Wiley and Sons, 1985.

Glover, J. *Causing Death and Saving Lives*. Harmondsworth, England: Penguin, 1977.

Glover, Jacqueline J. and Cindy H. Rushton. From Baby Doe to Baby K: Evolving challenges in pediatric ethics. *Journal of Law, Medicine and Ethics* (1995) 23:1, 5–6.

Goldberg, A. B. *In the matter of Baby K*, Letters to the Editor, *Journal of Law, Medicine & Ethics* (1995): 23:3, 300.

Goldenring, John. The brain-life theory: Towards a consistent biological definition of humanness. *Journal of Medicine Ethics* (1985): 11:2, 198–204.

Goldhagen, D. *Hitler's Willing Executioners*. New York: Knopf, 1996.

Gottlieb, Lawrence, and Mark J. Zucker. Organs for undocumented aliens? A transplantation dilemma. *Cambridge Quarterly of Healthcare Ethics* (1995): 4:2, 231.

Gould, Peter. The tyranny of taxonomy. *The Sciences* (May/June 1982): 7–9.

Gould, Stephen J. *The Mismeasure of Man*. New York: W. W. Norton, 1981.

———. *Dinosaur in a Hay Stack* New York: Harmony Books, 1995.

Graf Haber, Joram. Review of Peter Singer. Rethinking life and death. *Cambridge Quarterly of Healthcare Ethics* (1996): 5:1, 311–15.

Graves, Florence G. Writing for his life. *American Journalism Review* (March 1997): 25–31.

Gutmann, Amy, and Dennis Thompson. *Democracy and Disagreement*. Cambridge, Mass.: Harvard University Press, 1996.

Habermas, Jürgen. *Moral Consciousness and Communicative Action*. Cambridge, Mass.: MIT Press, 1990.

———. *Justification and Application: Remarks on Discourse Ethics*. Cambridge, Mass.: MIT Press, 1993.

Hanley, Ruth. *In re T.A.C.P. Issues in Law and Medicine* (1993): 9:1, 65–68.

Hardwig, John. What about the family? *Hastings Center Report* (1990): 20:2, 5–10.

Harris, J. *The Value of Life*. London: Routledge, 1985.

Hauptman, Paul, and Kevin J. O'Connor. Medical progress: Procurement and allocation of solid organs for transplantation. *New England Journal of Medicine* (February 6, 1997): 226:6, 422–31.

Henton, Darcy. "Wasted" transplants under fire in Alberta. *Toronto Star*, April 7, 1995, A10.

Hoppe, Arthur. Mickey Mantle's lucky liver. *San Francisco Chronicle*, June 16, 1995, A29.

Horgan, John. Eugenics revisited. *Scientific American*, (June 1993): 122–31.

Hubert, Cynthia. Transplant pioneer loses battle for life. *Sacramento Bee*, May 25, 1997.

Hughes, James J. Brain Death and Technological Change: Personal Identity, Neural Prostheses and Uploading. Second International Symposium on Brain Death. Havana, Cuba, February 27–March 1, 1995.

In re Conservatorship of Wanglie, No. PX-91–283 (Minn. Dist. Ct.) Prob. Div., July 1, 1991.

In re T.A.C.P. 609 So. 2d 588 (Fl. 1992).

In the Matter of Baby K 832 F. Supp. 1022 (Va. 1993), 1029.

Jameton, Andrew. *Nursing Practice: The Ethical Issues*. Englewood Cliffs, N.J.: Prentice Hall, 1984, 24. In Daniel F. Chambliss, *Beyond Caring: Hospitals, Nurses, and the Social Organization of Ethics*. Chicago: University of Chicago Press, 1996, 138.

Jecker, Nancy S. Caring for "socially undesirable" patients. *Cambridge Quarterly of Healthcare Ethics* (1996): 5:4, 500–510.

Jonsen, Albert R. The birth of bioethics. *Hastings Center Report*, Special Supplement (November–December 1993), S1.

———. Casuistry: An alternative or complement to principles? *Kennedy Institute of Ethics Journal* (1995): 5:3, 237–51.

Katz, A. H., and D. M. Proctor. Social psychological characteristics of patients receiving hemodialysis treatment for chronic renal failure. Public Health Service, Kidney Disease Control Program, July 1969. Quoted in Nancy S. Jecker, Caring for "socially undesirable" patients. *Cambridge Quarterly of Healthcare Ethics* (1996): 5:4, 509.

Kittay, Eva F. and Diana T. Meyers. The justice position and the care perspective. In *Women and Moral Theory*, ed. Eva F. Kittay and Diana T. Meyers. Savage, M.: Rowman and Littlefield, 1987.

Klevit, Harvey D., et al. Prioritization of health care services: A progress report by the Oregon Health Services Commission. *Archives of Internal Medicine* (1991): 151, 912–16.

Koch, Tom. *A Place in Time: Care Givers for Their Elderly*. Westport Conn.: Praeger 1993.

———. The Canadian question: What's so great about intelligence? *Cambridge Quarterly of Healthcare Ethics* (1996): 5:2, 307–10.

———. Living versus dying "with dignity": A new perspective on the euthanasia debate. *Cambridge Quarterly of Healthcare Ethics* (1996): 5:1, 50–61.

———. Normative and prescriptive criteria: The efficacy of organ transplantation allocation protocols. *Theoretical Medicine* (1996): 17:1, 75–93.

Koch, Tom, and Mark Ridgley. Distanced perspectives: Aids, Anencephaly, and AHP. *Theoretical Medicine and Bioethics* (1998): 19:1, 47–58.

Koch, Tom, and Mary Rowell. A pilot study on transplant eligibility criteria: Valuing the stories in numbers. *Pediatric Nursing* (1997): 23:2, 160–66.

Kolata, Gina. Transplants, morality and Mickey Mantle. *New York Times*, June 11, 1995.

————. In shift, prospects for survival will decide liver transplants. *New York Times*, November 15, 1996, A1, A26.

Kuczewski, Mark. Review of Jonathan D. Moreno. *Deciding Together: Bioethics and Moral Consensus. Cambridge Quarterly of Healthcare Ethics* (1997): 6: 3, 358–59.

Kuhse, Helga, and Peter Singer. *Should the Baby Live? The Problem of Handicapped Infants.* Oxford: Oxford University Press, 1985.

Lantos, John. Baby Doe five years later: Implications for child health. *New England Journal of Medicine* (1987): 317, 444–47.

————. Seeking justice for Priscilla. *Cambridge Quarterly of Healthcare Ethics* (1996): 5:4, 489.

Lefebvre, A., and E. Arndt. Working with facially disfigured children: A challenge in prevention. *Canadian Journal of Psychiatry* (1988): 33, 453–58.

Lewontin, R. C. *Biology as Ideology.* (New York: Harper Collins, 1993), 88.

Lomasky, Loren E. *Persons, Rights, and the Moral Community.* (New York: Oxford University Press, 1987).

Masson, J. M. *When Elephants Weep: The Emotional Lives of Animals.* New York: Delacorte Press, 1995.

McCurdy, David B. Alzheimer disease. *Making the Rounds in Health, Faith & Ethics.* Newsletter. Chicago: Parkridge Center, March 25, 1996, 5.

McKnight, J. Two tools for well-being: Health systems and communities. *Annals of Preventive Medicine.* Supplement: *Medicine in the 21st Century: Challenges in Personal and Public Health Promotion* (1994): 10:3, 23–26.

McPhee, John. *Levels of the Game.* Toronto: Macfarlane, Walter & Ross, 1969.

Minow, Martha, and Elizabeth V. Spelman. In context 63. *Southern California Law Review* (1990): 1597, 1632–33.

Moreno, Jonathan D. *Deciding Together: Bioethics and Moral Consensus.* New York: Oxford University Press, 1995.

Morowitz, Harold J. *The Facts of Life: Science & the Abortion Controversy.* New York: Oxford University Press, 1992.

Morreim, E. H. *Balancing Act: The New Medical Ethics of Medicine's New Economics.* Dodrecht and Boston: Kluwer Academic Publications, 1991.

Nelson, Hilde Lindemann. Dethroning choice: Analogy, personhood, and the new reproductive technologies. *Journal of Law, Medicine, and Ethics* (1995): 23:2, 129–35.

Nelson, James Lindemann. Taking families seriously. *Hastings Center Report* (1992): 22:4, 6–12.

Oberman, Michelle. Minor rights and wrongs. *Journal of Law, Medicine & Ethics* (1996): 24:2, 127–38.

Oksenberg, A. R. *The Identities of Persons*. Berkeley: University of California Press, 1975.

Olbrisch, M. E., and J. L. Levenson. Psychosocial evaluation of heart transplant candidates: An international survey of process, criteria, and outcomes. *Journal of Heart Lung Transplant* (1991): 10, 948–55.

Olson, D. *Decision Aids for Selection Problems*. New York: Springer, 1996.

Osorio, R. S. et al. Predicting recidivism after orthotopic liver transplantation for alcoholic liver disease. *Hematology* (1994): 20:1:1, 105–10.

Ott, Barbara B. Commentary on Tom Koch and M. Rowell. Changes in liver transplantation policy. *Pediatric Nursing* (1997): 23:2, 167–68.

Perkins, Henry S. Commentary: Distributing American hearts for transplantation: The predicament of living in the global village. *Cambridge Quarterly of Healthcare Ethics* (1995): 4:2, 232–36.

Pernick, Martin S. *The Black Stork: Eugenics and the Death of "Defective" Babies in American Medicine and Motion Pictures Since 1915*. New York: Oxford University Press, 1995.

Post, Stephen G. *The Moral Challenge of Alzheimer Disease*. Baltimore: Johns Hopkins University Press, 1995.

———. Baby K: Medical futility and the free exercise of religion. *Journal of Law, Medicine & Ethics* (1995): 23:1, 21.

Price, David P. Contemporary transplant initiatives: Where's the harm in them? *Journal of Law, Medicine & Ethics* (1996): 24:2, 242.

Quill, Timothy E., and Gerrit Kimsma. End-of-life care in the Netherlands and the United States: A comparison of values, justifications, and practices. *Cambridge Quarterly of Healthcare Ethics* (1997): 6:2, 189–204.

Rabiner, D., and J. Coie. Effect of expectancy indications on rejected children's acceptance by unfamiliar peers. *Developmental Psychology* (1989): 25, 450–57.

Ramos, E. L., et al. The evaluation of candidates for renal transplantation: The current practice of U.S. transplant centers. *Transplantation* (1994): 57, 490–97.

Raphael, David. *Moral Philosophy*. Oxford: Oxford University Press, 1981.

Rawls, John. *A Theory of Justice*. Cambridge, Mass.: Harvard University Press, 1971.

———. *Political Liberalism*. New York: Columbia University Press, 1993.

Reeve, Christopher. *Still Me: A Life*. New York: Random House, 1998.

Reilly, Philip R. *The Surgical Solution: A History of Involuntary Sterilization in the United States*. Baltimore: Johns Hopkins University Press, 1991.

Remnick, D. Reading Japan. *New Yorker*, February 6, 1995, 38–43.

Rescher, Nicholas. *Pluralism: Against the Demand for Consensus*. New York: Oxford University Press, 1993.

Roe v. Wade 410 US 113 (1973).

Rosenbaum, P. L., and R. W. Armstrong. Self-perceived social function among disabled children in regular classrooms. *Developmental and Behavioral Pediatrics* (1992): 13:1, 11–16.

Russell, Sabin. Livers for transplant can show up quickly. *San Francisco Chronicle*, June 9, 1995, A6.

Rymer, Russ. A silent childhood, II. *New Yorker*, April 20, 1992, 67–69.

Sacks, Oliver. *Awakenings*. 1973; London: Pan Books, 1982.

———. *The Man Who Mistook His Wife for a Hat*. New York: Summit Books, 1985.

———. *An Anthropologist on Mars*. New York: Knopf, 1995.

Saaty, Thomas L. *The Analytic Hierarchy Process*. New York: McGraw-Hill, 1980.

———. An exposition of the AHP to the paper, "Remarks on the Analytic Hierarchy Process." *Management Science* (1990): 36, 259–68.

———. *Fundamentals of Decision Making and Priority Theory with the Analytic Hierarchy Process*. Pittsburgh: RWS Publications, 1994.

Saaty, Thomas L., and Joyce M. Alexander. *Conflict Resolution: The Analytic Hierarchy Process*. New York: Praeger, 1989.

Saaty, Thomas L., and Luis G. Vargas. *Decision Making in Economic, Political, Social and Technological Environments*. AHP Series Vol. 7. Pittsburgh, PA: RWS Publications, 1994.

Schneider, Karen S., and Jane Shapiro. Local hero, *People Magazine*, January 27, 1997, 82–86.

Schneiderman, Lawrence J., and Sharyn Manning. *The Baby K Case*: A search for the elusive standard of medical care. *Cambridge Quarterly of Healthcare Ethics* (1997): 6:1, 9–18.

Silberstein, L. J. *Martin Buber's Social and Religious Thought*. New York: New York University Press, 1989.

Singer, Peter. *Rethinking Life and Death: The Collapse of Our Traditional Ethics*. New York: St. Martin's Press, 1995.

Solomon, Mildred Z. From what's neutral to what's meaningful: Reflections on a study of medical interpreters. *The Journal of Clinical Ethics* (1997): 8:1, 88–93.

Somerville, Margaret A. Genetics, reproductive technologies, euthanasia, and the search for a new societal paradigm. *Social Science and Medicine* (1996): 42:12, ix–xii.

———. Euthanasia by confusion. *UNSW Law Journal* (1997): 20:13, 1–20.

Spielman, B. Collective decisions about medical futility. *Journal of Law, Medicine & Ethics* (1995): 22:2, 152–60.

Spike, Jeffery, and Jane Greenlaw. Ethics consultation: Persistent brain death and religion: Must a person believe in death to die? *Journal of Law, Medicine & Ethics* (1995): 23:3, 20–23.

Starzl, Thomas E., et al. A multifactorial system for equitable selection of cadaver kidney recipients. *Journal of the American Medical Association* (1987): 257: 22, 3073–75.

Startzl, T. E., et al. Equitable allocation of extrarenal organs: With special reference to the liver. *Transplantation Proceedings* (1988): 20:1, 131–38.

Stupf, David A. The infant with anencephaly. *New England Journal of Medicine* (1990): 322, 669.

Sudnow, D. *Passing On*. Englewood Cliffs, N.J.: Prentice Hall, 1967.

Sytsma, S. E. Anencephalics as organ sources. *Theoretical Medicine* (1996): 17:1, 19–32.

Taylor, Alan D. *Mathematics and Politics: Strategy, Voting, Power, and Proof*. New York: Springer-Verlag, 1997.

Taylor, Charles. *The Ethics of Authenticity*. Cambridge, Mass.: Harvard University Press, 1992.

Ten Have, Henk A. Medical technology assessment and ethics—Ambivalent relations. *Hastings Center Report* (1995): 25:5, 13–19.

Tesh, S. *Hidden Arguments: Political Ideology and Disease Prevention Policy*. New Brunswick, N.J.: Rutgers University Press, 1988.

Thomas, Lewis. *The Fragile Species*. New York: Collier Books, 1992, 26.

Thomasma, David. Anencephalics as organ donors. In *Biomedical Ethics Reviews–1989*, ed. James M. Humber and Robert F. Almeder. Clifton, N.J.: Humana Press, 1990.

———. An analysis for and against euthanasia and assisted suicide. Part 1. *Cambridge Quarterly of Healthcare Ethics* (1996): 5:1, 62–76.

———. Commentary: Guidelines for rationing resemble process of family decision making. Commentary on the Asbury draft policy. *British Medical Journal* (1996): 312:7045, 1531–32.

Thomasma, David, and Thomasine Kushner, eds. *Birth to Death: Science and Ethics*. New York: Cambridge University Press, 1996.

Tribe, Laurence H. *Abortion: The Clash of Absolutes*. New York: W. W. Norton & Co., 1990.

Van Leeuwen, Evert, and Gerrit K. Kimsma. Acting or letting go: Medical decision making in neonatology in the Netherlands. *Cambridge Quarterly of Heathcare Ethics* (1993): 2, 265–69.

Veatch, Robert M. Should basic care get priority? Doubts about rationing the Oregon way. *Kennedy Institute of Ethics Journal* (1991): 1:3, 187–206.

———. Research on "big ticket" items: Ethical implications for equitable access. *Journal of Law, Medicine & Ethics* (1994): 22:2, 148–51.

Wackers, G. L. *Constructivist Medicine*. Maastricht, Holland: Universitaire Pers Maastricht, 1994.

Walters, James W. Proximate personhood as a standard for making difficult treatment decisions: Imperiled newborns as a case study. *Bioethics* (1992): 6: 1, 12–22.

Walzer, Michael. *Spheres of Justice: A Defense of Pluralism and Equality*. Oxford: Basil Blackwell, 1983, 31.

———. *Thick and Thin: Moral Argument at Home and Abroad*. Notre Dame, Ind.: Notre Dame University Press, 1994.

White, M., and J. Gribbin. *Stephen Hawking: A Life in Science*. New York: Penguin Books, 1992.

Wolf, Susan M. Shifting paradigms in bioethics and health law: The rise of a new pragmatism. *American Journal of Law and Medicine* (1994): 20:4, 395–415.

Wright, R. *The Moral Animal*. New York: Pantheon Books, 1994.

York, G. Y., R. M. Ballarno, and R. O. York. Baby Doe regulations and medical judgment. *Social Science and Medicine* (1990): 30, 657–64.

Young, Jenny M., Carolyn L. Marshall, and Elizabeth J. Anderson. Amyotrophic lateral sclerosis patients' perspectives on use of mechanical ventilation. *Health and Social Work* (1994): 19:4, 253–60.

Young, Jenny M., and Paule McNicoll. Against all odds: Positive life experiences of persons with advanced amyotrophic Lateral Sclerosis. *Health and Social Work* (1998): 23:1, 35–43.

Index

About the Author

TOM KOCH is a researcher and writer specializing in the care of the fragile and their caregivers. He is the author of eight other books, including *Mirrored Lives: Aging Children and Elderly Parents* (Praeger, 1990) and *A Place in Time: Caregivers for Their Elderly* (Praeger, 1993).